GASTRIC SLEEVE

Bariatric Cookbook
for beginners

Easy and Nutritional Recipes to Lose Weight Fast and Stay
Healthy for Every Stage of Bariatric Surgery Recovery

Ashley Evans

Content

1   Introduction

Part I

3   Chapter 1: **All About Bariatric Surgery**

9   Chapter 2: **A New Way of Life**

15   Chapter 3: **Your Diet After Bariatric Surgery**

Part II

38   Chapter 4: **Full Liquid Diet**

46   Chapter 5: **Puréed Foods**

55   Chapter 6: **Soft Foods**

64   Chapter 7: **Breakfast**

73   Chapter 8: **Sides and Snacks**

81   Chapter 9: **Vegetarian Dinners**

92   Chapter 10: **Fish and Seafood Dinners**

100   Chapter 11: **Poultry Dinners**

108   Chapter 12: **Pork and Beef Dinners**

116   Chapter 13: **Sweets and Treats**

124   Chapter 14: **Dressings, Sauces, and Seasonings**

130   *Appendix 1: Measurement Conversion Chart*

131   *Appendix 2: Recipe Index*

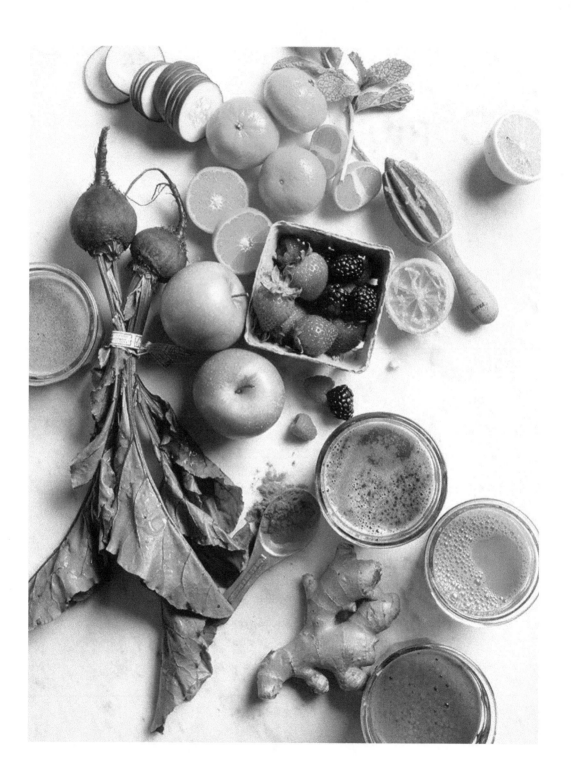

Introduction

I have been invested in finding ways to successfully lose weight and keep it off since I can remember. Having struggled with my weight from a young age, I'm no stranger to yo-yo dieting. In my search for the perfect diet, I have come across various natural ways to lose weight—the Mediterranean diet being a firm favorite. But, the fact of the matter is not everyone can do this the natural way. Some people need help, and nothing presses the weight reset button as hard as bariatric surgery.

It's frequently someone's last desperate attempt to take their life and health back. Fortunately, the success rate of getting a gastric sleeve or bypass is high, so you get a second chance at life.

With that being said, surgery is not where this process ends. Weight-loss surgery is a life-changing procedure, which you will need to adapt to. You will have to change your relationship with food entirely. Gone are the days of using food as a method to celebrate achievements or suppress emotions. You won't be eating because you're bored or lonely, but to fuel your body efficiently.

The size of your new stomach will only be a fraction of what it used to be, and can only handle a small portion of food at a time. This makes what you put into your mouth extra important, and I want to help you feed your body with only the best, most delicious food available.

In this cookbook, I will walk you through the various types of bariatric surgery, but the focus will be on vertical sleeve gastrectomy since it is considered the safest yet still effective weight-loss surgery out of all four methods.

But what I'm most excited about is helping you navigate your new way of life, and assisting you in leaving behind any fear you might have surrounding bariatric surgery. I also can't wait to walk you through the bariatric transition diet and help you set up your kitchen to ensure long-term success.

Of course, what would a cookbook be without the cooking? I am proud of the selection of sleeve-friendly recipes that are included in this book. They're formatted to include the right balance of protein, carbohydrates, and fat. I've done all the math so you can just decide on the meal and prepare it knowing you'll experience no discomfort after. All meals are based on the bariatric diet and curated to exclude foods that upset your stomach.

I hope this cookbook will help you settle into life after weight-loss surgery with less anxiety while offering you some form of comfort (food) within the confines of the post-op diet.

Chapter 1: All About Bariatric Surgery

B ariatric surgical procedures are often the only hope for those that are severely obese. It works by inhibiting the amount of food a person can eat and limiting the calories they will consume per day. The fewer calories a person eats in relation to what their body needs to function, the more weight they will lose.

The most common weight-loss surgeries are gastric bypass, vertical sleeve gastrectomy (VSG), adjustable gastric band, and biliopancreatic diversion with duodenal switch (BPD/DS). All of these are done laparoscopically, which means they are minimally invasive, and the hospital stay won't be too long.

4 Types of Bariatric Procedures

Gastric Bypass (Roux-en-Y)

The first component of the procedure is separating the stomach into two sections. The small pouch connected to the esophagus will be approximately one ounce in volume and will continue to receive food. Food will no longer reach the bottom part of the stomach. Next, a section of the small intestine is disconnected and reconnected to the small part of the stomach. This means food will be re-routed directly from the stomach to the remaining intestine.

The procedure works on the same premise as most other weight-loss surgeries: the significant reduction of the stomach's size means only a small amount of food can be accommodated at a time, which translates to lower calorie intake. The fact that a part of the small intestine—which also absorbs calories—no longer has food going through it also decreases the absorption of nutrients and thus calories.

- The procedure is performed laparoscopically.
- Usually a three-day hospital stay.
- Two to four weeks of restricted activity post-op.
- Non-reversible.

Vertical Sleeve Gastrectomy

A VSG is where up to 80 percent of a person's stomach is removed by stapling and dividing it vertically. A banana-shaped section of the stomach remains. It works for the same reason that gastric bypass does—limited stomach capacity. A person isn't able to eat large portions, and this leads to reduced calorie intake.

In addition, VSG seems to affect gut hormones that play a role in hunger, satiety and stabilizing blood sugar levels (Ionut et al., 2013).

- The procedure is performed laparoscopically.
- Two-day hospital stay.
- Two to three weeks of restricted activity post-op.
- Non-reversible.
- Weight-loss results are similar to that of gastric bypass surgery, but the long-term maintenance of the weight loss is up to 50 percent higher (Richardson et al., 2009).

Adjustable Gastric Band

Often just called "the band," this procedure involves a silicone ring being placed around the top part of the stomach to create a small pouch. The size of the opening between the pouch and the more substantial part of the stomach can be adjusted. If the opening is big, the feeling of fullness after eating won't be nearly as much as when the opening is smaller.

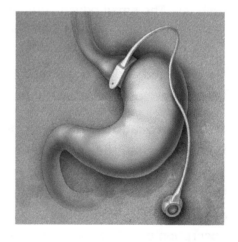

To reduce the size of the opening, sterile saline is injected through a port placed under the person's skin. Similarly, the opening can be enlarged by withdrawing the liquid. This process is done gradually over time to achieve the ideal tightness.

The idea is that the band will restrict how much food can be eaten at any time combined with the slow speed at which it passes through the band leads to weight loss. However, some studies have challenged this notion, claiming that food passes through the band quickly, which means patients don't feel satiated for longer (Seeras et al., 2020).

- The procedure is done laparoscopically.
- Hospital stay is less than 24 hours.
- Involves no cutting or re-routing.
- Is reversible.
- Is the least effective of all the bariatric procedures.

Biliopancreatic Diversion with Duodenal Switch (BPD/DS)

The BPD/DS is similar to gastric bypass surgery except for two variances. The section of the small intestine that is bypassed is significantly larger. In addition, the food only mixes with the bile and pancreatic enzymes far down the small intestine resulting in minimal absorption of calories and nutrients.

It is usually done in two stages to minimize the risk of having a lengthy procedure. First, the doctor will do a VSG. Twelve to 18 months later, the bypass part of the process will be completed.

- The procedure is done either laparoscopically or as traditional open surgery.
- Hospital stay is up to three days.
- Non-reversible.
- A person will need to take vitamin and mineral supplements daily.
- Although it is the most effective of all bariatric surgeries, it is high risk and can cause long-term health problems.

Since the weight loss after the VSG part of the BPD/DS is so significant, doctors decided that sleeve gastrectomy is efficient enough to see results—with less risk and complications. Let's have a closer look at the advantages and disadvantages of the sleeve.

People who've had sleeve surgery lose up to 60-70% of excess weight.

Here is a breakdown of the common trend of weight loss:

- In the first two weeks, most people will lose around one pound a day. You can expect to drop anywhere from 10 to 20 pounds.
- In the first three months, expect a 35-45% reduction of weight.
- In the first six months, people lost up to 60% of any excess weight, and after a year, up to 70%.

This is impressive, considering that there's no need for foreign objects or re-routing of any kind.

But there are more advantages than just losing weight. You will also improve many weight-related health problems (Hoyuela, 2017).

These include:

- Type 2 diabetes
- Fatty liver disease
- Hypertension
- High cholesterol
- PCOS
- Infertility
- Sleep apnea
- And non-weight-related issues such as asthma, migraines, depression, and urinary incontinence.

VSG also removes the part of the stomach that produces Ghrelin—a hormone that stimulates hunger.

Then there's dumping syndrome—the discomfort so many bariatric patients experience when they overeat or consume sugary foods (Mayo Clinic, n.d.). Well, VSG is avoided or, at the very least, minimized since the opening of the stomach stays intact.

Compared to other bariatric surgeries, the drawbacks are minor. The main shortcoming is, strangely enough, one of the advantages—dumping syndrome. Since someone who has undergone VSG won't experience any discomfort after eating sugary foods, they'll be likely to continue consuming them. As you can imagine, this will significantly reduce any weight loss.

There's also a chance of gastric leaks and other complications related to stapling. As with other weight-loss surgery, the potential of vitamin deficiency exists, but can easily be overcome by drinking supplements daily.

After analyzing the pros and cons of gastric sleeve surgery, it's clear why doctors recommend this procedure over other bariatric surgeries. The disadvantages are few, and the advantages when compared to other methods make VSG the superior choice. However, many people are torn between gastric bypass and sleeve surgery since the bypass procedure has slightly more impressive weight loss results. But, before you make up your mind, let's compare the two.

Bypass vs. the Sleeve

These two procedures are very similar; although the methods differ, it's all about reducing the size of the stomach and decreasing the amount of food a person can consume. They're both effective tools to lose weight in the long-term and improve obesity-related conditions such as diabetes, high cholesterol, high blood pressure, etc.

The gastric sleeve is a less complicated surgery, taking between 40 and 70 minutes to complete, whereas bypass surgery can take up to three hours.

Furthermore, gastric bypass patients may experience short-term complications such as bowel obstruction, ulcers, and internal hernias. The chance of sleeve patients developing any of these is close to zero.

If dietary constraints are the deciding factor for you, the changes you'll have to make will be the same for bypass and sleeve surgery. The main difference will be how much you can eat. If you opt for the gastric sleeve surgery, your stomach pouch will be able to hold up to three ounces. On the other hand, the gastric bypass will leave you with a stomach the size of a golf ball, which equates to 1 ounce.

Any decision of what bariatric surgery method to select should be made alongside your doctor. They will consider things like your age, overall health, weight, and expectations when making a decision. For example, gastric bypass surgery will usually be selected for patients with a Body Mass Index over 45, and not VSG.

Common Misconceptions

Before we move on to life after bariatric surgery, I think it is important to dispel some common myths about weight-loss surgery.

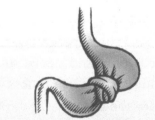

≫ **It's the easy way out.** If you're expecting a magic bullet, you won't get one. Although surgery will make your weight-loss journey significantly more manageable, you will still need to put in a lot of hard work and dedication.

≫ **It doesn't work in the long run.** Many people believe that surgery isn't a long-term solution since most people regain weight. Research shows that, compared to people who lost weight naturally, bariatric patients lost more weight and maintained their results (Huang et al., 2016).

≫ **It isn't safe.** The surgery itself is safer than other standard surgical procedures, with the risk of death within the first 30 days following surgery as low as 0.13% (Sudan et al., 2014). The risk of death due to various comorbidities is also significantly reduced. For example, the diabetes mortality rate decreases by more than 90% after bariatric surgery.

Chapter 2: A New Way of Life

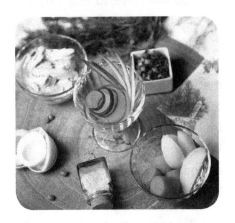

It doesn't matter what bariatric surgery method you end up choosing; it is a life-altering procedure. For it to be successful, you will need to approach life and your food choices differently. This may be more challenging than going through the actual surgery and recovery process. Here is how you will have to alter your outlook.

Before we get to your mindset, you will have to prepare those around you. You may even consider involving those closest to you in the process. This will make it easier to understand what exactly is happening and how they can best support you. Of course, you won't have to share your decision to have bariatric surgery with those who aren't part of your inner circle, or those who might only have negative things to say. Deciding to have surgery is personal, and I suggest you only discuss it with people you know will support and encourage you. If someone who you thought would be understanding turns out against it, don't let the comments dissuade you. It's usually because they are not understanding the process, or they are afraid of the unknown and what can happen.

Remind yourself that the only person you're held accountable for is yourself. Keep your head held high and surprise those who doubt you with a remarkable transformation!

Now, let's move on to you and your new way of life.

Eat Without Fear

You will have to learn how to eat again. After your surgery, you will first start consuming liquids and gradually move on to eat a balanced diet of almost all the foods you used to enjoy. In the beginning, you may feel a little overwhelmed with not 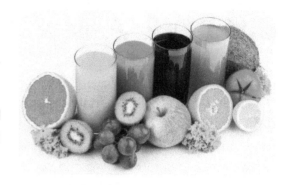 knowing what is safe to eat, and this fear may lead to you to avoid eating altogether. This is never a good idea; if you starve yourself, the chances of binging on the wrong foods is more likely.

Recognize that asking for help is okay. You need to rely on medical professionals to share with you any information that will put your fears at ease. They will tell you precisely what you should and shouldn't eat, which should put your mind at ease. You may also consider joining a bariatric support group where you can share what you're going through and get advice from people who've been where you are or who are currently struggling with the same thing. Support is paramount, especially in the early days when you are still finding your feet.

You may be scared that your old eating habits will come back and before you know it, you'll undo the benefits of the weight-loss surgery. This is the moment the negative thinking needs to be silenced—tell yourself this time is different. I know many people who get bariatric surgery do so because they have spent their whole lives yo-yo dieting, which is their last attempt at success. Well, weight-loss surgery gives you a great head start, which will be a massive help.

It will be difficult (near impossible) for you to slip back to the "old you" if you change your mindset to one of victory. Always keep in your mind that this is not "just another diet," it is a permanent lifestyle change. Commit to yourself!

Be Compassionate

Probably the most important thing you can do is to be kind to yourself—everything else will flow from it. Your self-talk directly affects your happiness, and this will influence how easy it will be for you to stick to these changes in the long run. To practice self-compassion, you have to be kind, mindful, and accept that you're only human.

Accept that all patients who undergo weight-loss surgery will make mistakes. The triumph lies in how you react to any slip-ups. If you're sympathetic with yourself instead of cruel and criticizing, the chances of sliding back into old habits are far less. Remember that we're all human; embrace your victories but your defeats, too. Leave no space for self-denigration when you do fail. Consider that maybe your mind just needed a break from constantly focusing on your goals. If you're afraid of this happening again, do something relaxing. Meditation is a great way to quiet the mind and maintain perspective.

Whatever the reasons behind any blunders, don't fixate on them—move on and get excited about your future.

Learn New Eating Habits

It will be necessary for you to adjust the way you eat, especially just after surgery, as your body gets used to this change. But it goes further than that, and you will have to change your relationship with food entirely for long-term success. Some doctors may even suggest you see a therapist to help you understand why you were overweight in the first place. If you're like me, you eat when you're bored, stressed, or sad. The only thing I found that could snap me out of this behavior was to see someone who gave me the tools to overcome the unhealthy connection I had with food.

It's difficult—in society today, food plays such a central role—almost all celebrations are around food of some sort. This is why it is extra vital for you to take back your power and stop letting food take control. For example, if you're an emotional eater, learn healthy ways to cope with your feelings without using food as a distraction. If you always eat when you're lonely, why not call a friend if you'd like some company? Food is not your friend; it is fuel for your body.

There are various ways you can shift the emphasis from eating to some or other activity. Instead of meeting friends for dinner, why not plan a day to meet up and exercise or go hiking? If you give food less of a fundamental role in life, it will lose its grip.

Here are three tips to keep you on track.

1. **Stick to the Basics**

Be mindful of the fact that it is going to take some time for you to understand the dos and don'ts of your new diet. The most crucial time is the first few weeks after surgery. You will have to stick to the rules to not get sick. It's not a matter of ifs or buts. After the initial transition period, you'll be able to eat normally. But always keep in mind that overeating is not what you should ever aim for—not only will you feel ill, you'll be working against your body and the weight-loss surgery. Keep the basics of the bariatric diet in mind, and that way, you'll know exactly what your stomach's limits are and what foods you can have.

2. **Beat the Cravings**

Regrettably, for many people who've struggled with weight throughout their life, giving in to cravings is like flipping an 'on' switch. Telling yourself that you'll eat only one Oreo usually turns into an entire sleeve or box. This binge-type behavior snowballs into disappointment and self-hate, which can lead to more binging. Instead of giving in immediately, stop, and check your motives. When you do decide it is worth giving in to your cravings, try to manage your actions. You don't want it to spiral and you end up overindulging the entire weekend.

3. Stop Eating When You're Full

Your body will tell you when it has had enough, and it is up to you to listen and resist taking another bite. If you practice mindful eating, it will be much easier to stop when you've had enough. I suggest you turn off the TV and remove any distractions that take your attention away from eating. A lot of the time, we're so focused on an episode of our favorite show that we forget we're eating—it's a mechanical action. Before you know it, you've eaten more than your body can take, and you're left feeling bloated and nauseous.

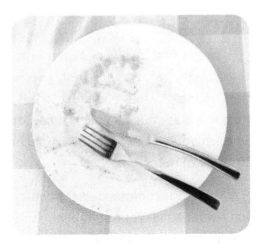

A huge part of your long-term success depends on your relationship with food. You must take away any control it has over you. Here are some tips to help you get started

- Find strategies that help you manage your emotions to stop emotional eating. Similarly, find ways to break the pattern of eating if you're in a bad mood.
- Go for a walk when you get a craving. They only last for 15 to 20 minutes, 30 at most, so if you can distract yourself for that span of time, you'll beat the urge to give in (Ledochowski et al., 2015).
- Always carry healthy snacks with you when you know you're going to have a busy day. This will prevent you from having to choose less-healthy options when you get peckish.
- It's a good idea to make a shopping list before you go to the grocery store. If you stick to buying only what is on the list, you will avoid impulse buying unhealthy food that doesn't fit in with your gastric diet.

How to Eat

For the first few weeks after surgery, how you eat will be just as important as what you eat. Besides that, you will have to be conscious of the size of the bites you take when you start to eat normally again. Considering that your stomach is so much smaller, it can only tolerate a certain amount of food at a time, so you will have to take smaller bites, chew up to 30 times, and eat for 20 to 30 minutes.

It's also recommended that you don't drink anything while you eat. You don't want to fill your stomach with liquid instead of food. There's also a possibility that fluid will flush food out of your stomach too quickly.

Another issue you will face is forcing yourself to eat when you're not hungry. Since there is a massive reduction in the ghrelin—the hormone that promotes hunger—you won't have an appetite. But you must meet your protein and nutrient needs. I suggest setting alarms throughout the day to remind you to eat when you're not hungry. Since your stomach is so small, you may need to eat up to six times a day to get all the nutrients you need.

To prepare yourself for all these changes, you can start learning these new habits even before surgery. You can also follow the recipes in this cookbook so long to get used to eating a bariatric diet.

Here are some small ways you can start to form sleeve-friendly eating habits.

1. Downsize your plates and bowls.
2. Teach yourself to take smaller bites.
3. Chew your food at least 25 times before swallowing.
4. Don't inhale your food. Eat slowly.
5. Stop eating when you're full. A sigh, burp, hiccup, and even a runny nose may signal that your body has had enough.

Chapter 3: Your Diet After Bariatric Surgery

I'm going to guess that you are very familiar with various weight-loss diets. You've probably tried all of them but failed to stick to it for whatever reason. The decision to have VSG isn't made overnight and usually comes after years of trying and failing to lose weight. So, you most likely are familiar with the way diets work and the nutritional benefits of specific foods. This counts to your advantage while adapting to a bariatric diet.

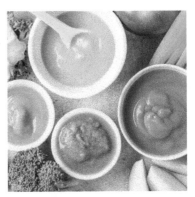

VSG Nutrition

You don't need to be a dietician or a nutrition expert to understand the eating plan I will share in this cookbook. There are some basic principles you need to keep in mind, and that's it! The recipes you'll find in this book take each of these considerations into account for your convenience. But let's first look at how the macronutrients (protein, fat, carbohydrates) will need to be adapted to the bariatric diet.

Protein

Protein is the most important macronutrient following surgery. Protein gives you energy and will preserve your muscles as you lose weight. It also takes longer to break down than carbohydrates, so that you will feel satiated for longer. It is also less calorie-dense than fat, which means, out of all the macronutrients, protein is the best post-op. The first two weeks after surgery, you won't be eating protein solids but will instead drink protein-rich smoothies. Later on, there will be a bigger mix of meals. This makes this cookbook invaluable as it will give you a variety of ideas while keeping your protein needs in mind.

Eating enough protein will also make your body heal from surgery faster. It is recommended that you consume between 2.11 to 3.52 ounces of protein a day based on ideal body weight. Counting how much protein you eat is the only way to make sure all your needs are being met. You can use an online food tracking app if you like to do things electronically. If you're old-school and prefer doing it by hand, here's a handy table of protein-rich foods, the recommended portion sizes, and the protein per ounce.

Protein Sources	Portion Size	Protein (ounces)*
Beek, pork, poultry, fish	2 ounces	0.49
Scallops, shrimp	3 ounces	0.63
Turkey, ham, roast beef, chicken, or other lunch meat	2 ounces	0.35
Eggs	1 large	0.24
Egg whites	2 large	0.28
Fat-free, 1% or 2% cottage or ricotta cheese	½ cup	0.49
Cheddar, mozzarella, Swiss, and other natural cheese	1 ounce	0.24
Non-fat Greek yogurt	6 ounces (3/4 cup)	0.52
Lentils (cooked)	½ cup	0.31
Beans (cooked)	½ cup	0.31
Avoid: High-fat foods such as cream, whole milk, fatty cuts of beef or pork, and skin on poultry.		

*   **Always check the label on foods as protein content may vary.**

If you find it difficult to reach sufficient protein levels, you can use protein shakes, powders, or bars.

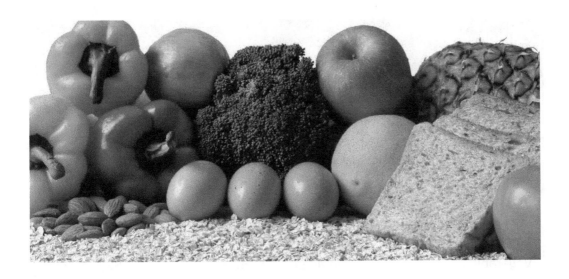

Carbohydrates

Although protein should be your main focus, carbohydrates are a quick energy source and are vital in various metabolic functions. The first few weeks after surgery, you will eat little to no carbs. Your body will instead metabolize fat stores and use the protein you eat as a fuel source.

When you do reintroduce carbohydrates into your diet, remember that not all carbs are created equal. You get simple and complex carbs. The simple type is digested faster than complex carbs, which leads to a blood sugar spike that isn't good for your overall health and weight loss goals. Foods containing white refined flour, a lot of sugar, and are highly processed are considered simple carbs.

On the bariatric diet, you will consume only complex carbohydrates such as whole-grain foods, fruits, and veggies. These foods are rich in fiber, vitamins, and minerals and break down slower, preventing unnecessary fluctuating blood sugar levels.

Once you're allowed to eat normally, you should aim to eat 35 to 45 percent of your daily calories in carbohydrates.

Carbohydrate Sources	Portion Size	Carbohydrate (ounces)
Fresh fruit	1 serving = ½ cup Recommended: 2 to 3 servings per day after initial liquid and soft food diet.	1.58
Vegetables	1 serving = 1 cup Recommended: 4 servings per day after initial liquid and soft food diet.	0.52
Oatmeal	½ cup	0.49
Whole-grain bread	1 slice	0.52
Brown or white rice	½ cup	0.81
Whole-wheat pasta	1/3 cup	0.98
Barley	1/3 cup	0.81
Ancient grains (quinoa, millet, spelt, farrow)	1/3 cup	0.52
Avoid: Refined grains, cookies, cakes, pastries, candies, fruit juice, and soda.		

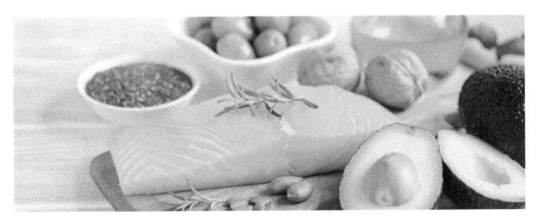

Fats

You will have to keep an eye on your fat intake since it is such a calorie-dense food—overeat fat, and you'll stall your weight loss. That doesn't mean you shouldn't eat it at all. We need dietary fat to help absorb fat-soluble vitamins like A, D, E, and K.

There are two types of fat; saturated and unsaturated. Saturated fat should be limited as it can increase your cholesterol and chances of a heart attack. Processed foods, coconut oil, full-fat dairy, butter, beef, pork, and chicken contain saturated fat.

Unsaturated fat comes from nuts, seeds, and olives. Fish is also a good source of these healthy fats. To lower your cholesterol levels and reduce your risk of heart disease, unsaturated fat is your friend.

Keep an eye on food labels of processed foods. These products may claim to be fat-free or low fat but usually contain hidden sugar or sodium to put some flavor back. Always choose low-fat or non-fat when it comes to dairy products, but opt for full-fat foods in the form of nuts, seeds, avocadoes, olives, and fatty fish.

In the beginning, you will consume minimal amounts of fat. However, in the long-term, you're looking at 30 percent of your daily calories from fats—less than 7 percent of this should be from saturated fats.

Fat Sources	Portion Sizes (one serving)	Fat (ounces)
Avocado	1 tablespoon	0.49
Chia	2 teaspoons	0.63
Olive oil	1 teaspoon	0.15
Almonds	6 tablespoons	0.12
Walnuts	2 tablespoons	0.18
Peanuts	10 tablespoons	0.17
Nut butters	2 teaspoons	0.17

Limit: Butter, palm and coconut oil, and full-fat dairy.

Avoid: Animal fats, fried foods, margarine containing trans fats, and food high in saturated fats.

Vitamins and Supplements

You will need to take a vitamin and mineral supplement for the rest of your life. If you're lucky, any deficiencies you have due to your gastric sleeve may disappear once you reach your goal weight, but it's best to err on the side of caution. You should follow up with your bariatric medical team on a regular basis to test your nutrients but never decide on your own to stop your supplementation.

Some of the most common deficiencies include:

Vitamin D: The recommended daily dosage is 3.000 IU, but it can be more, depending on the levels already in your blood.

Calcium: This is important for bone health—drink between 1.200 and 1.500 mg per day, divided into two or three doses.

Iron: Although it is not standard to recommend iron after weight-loss surgery, your doctor may do so your base-line levels are low.

Vitamin B12: Your doctor will routinely check your B12 levels. This vitamin is vital for normal nerve function and is regrettably usually impaired after VSG. You can either drink it as a daily supplement of 1.00 mcg per day or ask for an injection.

Some tips on drinking your supplements:

1. **Drink your vitamins close to mealtime.** A lot of vitamins are best absorbed with food.

2. **Don't use gummy vitamins.** They usually contain a lot of sugar, which means they're high in calories. Furthermore, most brands don't provide the 100 to 200 percent recommended daily allowance. If you prefer a chewable over liquid or pills, discuss it with your doctor and ask for a recommendation.

3. **Look for the USP verified symbol.** There are a lot of herbal supplements out there claiming to contain everything you need. Since the FDA doesn't regulate herbal medicines, there's no way for you to know if the claims they make are valid. Instead, look for USP-verified vitamins and minerals; that way, you know that you're getting high-quality products. You may also consider buying vitamins targeted for bariatric surgery patients. These supplements are usually more expensive, but they take the guesswork out of post-of bariatric supplementation.

Stay Hydrated

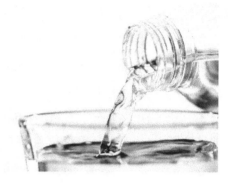

This will be your main focus after surgery, considering that dehydration is the most common complication (Ivanics, 2019). It will be challenging at first—a lot of us are used to enjoying a glass of water with our food, something you're not allowed to do after bariatric surgery. You won't be able to drink a large amount of fluid at once but will have to get into the habit of drinking small sips throughout the day.

I also suggest you take a more proactive approach and carry a water bottle with you. This way, you won't get stuck somewhere without access to water. You'll also be more conscious of how much you're drinking if you have a bottle in your hand where you can see the fluid getting less.

Fluid Sources: Water/Milk/Soy milk/Protein shakes/Decaffeinated coffee or tea/Non-carbonated, sugar-free drinks

It is recommended that you drink at least 64 ounces (eight cups) of fluids per day. You won't be able to meet this target straight after surgery, but this should be an achievable goal in the long-term.

Tips to help you stay hydrated:

- Drink a glass of water after waking up in the morning before you eat or drink anything else.
- Sip on a liquid between each small meal.
- Always carry a water bottle with you; stainless steel reusable is best!
- If you find

What about alcohol?

After VSG, your stomach's ability to process alcohol will be severely hindered. There is an enzyme in your stomach responsible for breaking down alcohol, and since most of your stomach has been removed, there is not enough meaning even a small amount will leave you intoxicated. Moreover, considering that your body mass is smaller than it was and the fact that you're only capable of ingesting small amounts of food, this will amplify the intoxication.

The fact that your blood-alcohol level will peak so much faster means the dehydration that follows drinking alcohol will also happen sooner than you expect.

With that being said, the answer to if you may drink alcohol after bariatric isn't exactly a n 'no.' You can indulge within moderation while keeping the above factors in mind. Ideally, you should wait three to 12 months after surgery before you drink anything alcoholic.

One last word of warning: transference addiction is a reality (Obesity Action Coalition, 2016). Patients who have a history of addiction may end up replacing their food addiction with other addictive behaviors, such as overconsumption of alcohol. If you notice any worrying changes in behavior, including excessive gambling, shopping, or other addictive behaviors, discuss it with your bariatric health team.

Some tips for drinking alcohol safely after bariatric surgery:

- Do not drink and eat at the same time.
- Consume low-calorie options and alcohol without added sugar. Whiskey on the rocks or red wine are good options.
- Avoid anything carbonated.
- Drink extra water when you are consuming alcohol.
- Eat a snack before you start drinking.

Keep Things Naturally Sweet

If you're used to eating the standard American diet, you'll know that your threshold for sweetness is higher than it was a few years ago. Everything is getting sugary and sweeter, making it more difficult to "kick the habit." The reality is that sugar is a drug, and we're always looking for our next fix (Avena et al., 2008).

VSG allows you to beat your sugar addiction. With this reset, you'll be able to jump start new eating habits. I'm not saying it will be easy, especially keeping in mind the pleasure centers in our brain that light up when we eat sugar. But, it is possible to retrain yourself to appreciate natural sweetness. Natural is full of candy; we just have to make the right decisions. Instead of reaching for a sugary dessert, you can eat some fresh berries. If your chocolate craving becomes overwhelming, add some 100 percent cocoa powder to a protein shake, and you have a delicious chocolate milkshake! The options are endless, and it's up to you to make the right choices.

When it comes to eating fruit, they contain many good, naturally occurring sugars your body likes. This is often forgotten since most sugars are lumped into one big category, so good sugars end up labeled as bad. The fact is that whole fruits have no added sugars. The phytochemicals and fiber content in fruit also delay the absorption of these natural sugars, meaning you won't experience any nasty blood sugar spikes as you would with refined sugar.

Just a few things to consider when it comes to eating fruit:

- Since protein is the most important macronutrient, eat it first, then fruits and vegetables, and other types of food.
- Fruit is high in calories, and carbohydrates, so don't overeat it, or you'll slow down your weight loss progress.

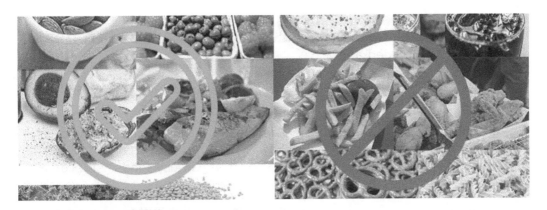

Foods to Avoid

Although the long-term goal is living as normal a life as possible, you will have to be mindful of what you put in your body. When you read up on VSG, you will see a lot of patients mention dumping syndrome. This is what happens when you eat foods you were supposed to avoid post-op. It's nothing to be scared of as it is entirely preventable. During the first three months after your VSG, there are foods you have to avoid. As time passes, you can slowly start reintroducing some of these foods into your diet, except for high-sugar and fried foods. These foods are known for causing dumping syndrome in not only bypass patients but also sleeve patients.

There are two types of dumping syndrome; early and late.

Early dumping syndrome will happen a short while after eating specific foods and is caused by the rapid emptying of the stomach. Symptoms include sweating, a rapid pulse, lightheadedness, a desire to lie down, nausea, and diarrhea. It is more common than late dumping and will pass as soon as the food has made its way out of your system.

Late dumping syndrome will only occur one to three hours after eating. You may feel shaky, dizzy, break out in cold sweats, experience confusion and anxiety, and feel hungry again. This is caused by hormonal changes caused by specific food and will pass when the food is out of your system.

Liquids	Proteins	Carbs	Fats	Other
Carbonated drinks	Breaded and deep-fried protein	Rice	Raw nuts and seeds	Asparagus stalks
Alcohol	Dry and tough meat	Pasta	Fried foods	Raw celery
Caffeine		Bread	Greasy foods	Coconut
Fruit juice		Dried fruits	Nut butter	Sweetened sauces or condiments
Sugary beverages		Skin of fruit		Cookies
		Fresh pineapple		Candy
		Popcorn		
		Granola and bran cereal		

Plan Your Meals

What is that saying again? "Failing to plan is planning to fail." This is very true when it comes to the long-term success of your VSG. Meal planning should form an integral part of your new lifestyle. If you take the time to map out your meals for the coming week—I don't mean down to every ingredient—you'll know if you have all the ingredients you need to prepare your meals.

It is particularly important in the days following surgery since you will have to keep an eye on your protein intake. By planning it all out, you can build your meals around protein and add fruit, vegetables, and grains.

Meal prep isn't limited to listing what you'll eat but includes pre-batching these meals. I am a big supporter of cooking meals for the week because you'll know there is a healthy meal waiting for you when you get home— removing any temptation of buying something unhealthy.

In essence, you'll be creating your own "frozen dinners," and you'll know exactly what's in them and that they're made according to the bariatric diet. In this cookbook, I include a lot of meals you can safely pre-cook, reheat, and eat.

Stock Your Kitchen

To cook mouth-watering sleeve-friendly meals, you need to stock up on some essentials—not just food but also some nifty must-have gadgets.

Food

You now know that the bariatric diet consists of protein, high-fiber carbs, and healthy fats, and can build your food stock around that. Make sure you have tons of different meats, fish and seafood, eggs, low-fat dairy, and legumes in your kitchen. You will also need some non-starchy vegetables, whole fruits, nuts and seeds, and various whole grains.

Here's a mini shopping list for when you first set up your bariatric kitchen.

- Almond flour
- Dried lentils
- Canned beans
- Dried spices and herbs
- Canned tuna, chicken, and salmon
- Eggs
- Olive oil
- Nuts and seeds

- Unsweetened pasta sauce
- Oats
- Whole wheat flour
- Low-sodium broth (vegetable, beef, and chicken)
- Frozen fruit
- Frozen vegetables
- Frozen meats
- Low- or no-fat dairy

If you still have food in your cupboard from your pre-VSG life, I suggest you donate anything that you can't use to a local food bank or a family in need.

Do a sweep of your kitchen, and if you see any of the following, clear it out.

- Boxed potatoes
- Bread
- Baked beans
- Cookies
- Chips
- Candy
- Cereal
- Crackers
- Frozen desserts

- Dried fruit
- High-carb frozen meals
- Sugary condiments
- High-fat products
- Refined pasta
- White rice
- Popcorn
- Caffeine

Gadgets

Who doesn't like a kitchen gadget that can make your life easier? You won't need fancy tools to prepare any of the meals in this cookbook—basic equipment such as knives, measuring cups, pots, and pans. There are a few tools I suggest you add to your kitchen to make cooking more comfortable and less time-consuming.

Mixer: It doesn't just mix, it whisks and can knead the dough.

Spiralizer and vegetable peeler: A very handy tool if you plan on making pasta dupes such as zucchini noodles. A peeler is essential as you will have to remove the skins from fruits and vegetables in the first few months after your surgery.

Immersion blender: Puree soup and sauces or other dishes while the pot or pan is still on the stove.

Muffin tin: You can use this to help with portion control.

Slow cooker: A great way to save time cooking.

Air fryer: Considering that you're not allowed to eat deep-fried food on the bariatric diet, air-fried food is the next best thing. You eat less than a teaspoon oil, and your food will come out nice and crispy.

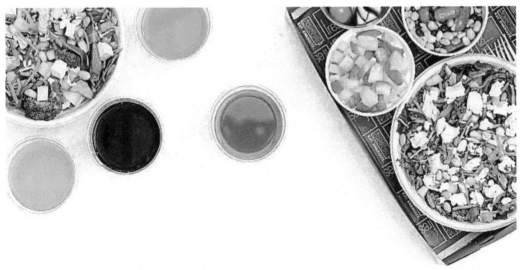

Your First 8 Weeks After Surgery

After sleeve surgery, your body will need time to get used to the new stomach. To help it along, your post-op diet will be divided into various textures starting with liquids, moving on to purées, then soft food, and eventually eating regular textured foods. Your doctor will determine how long you will stay in each phase, but I will share the general guidelines.

Week 1 and 2

These two weeks are all about getting and staying hydrated. As mentioned earlier, dehydration is the first complication post-op and can leave you feeling ill reasonably quickly. Weeks one and two will set the foundation and get you into the habit of drinking enough fluids daily—long after these two weeks have passed.

Here are some factors you will have to keep in mind during this time:

- Water comes first. Other clear liquids and any protein-rich shakes can be consumed after water. Try to drink at least 64 ounces of water a day.
- Shakes and smoothies shouldn't contain any seeds or pulp.
- Drink high-protein milk between meals to increase your protein consumption.

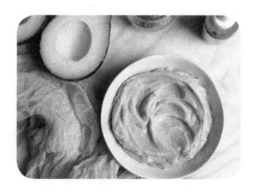

You will now be able to introduce soft, puréed food to your diet. Your body has done a lot of healing in the past two weeks, and the high protein-intake has helped significantly. Now it is more capable of absorbing nutrients and is reverting to proper digestion. The focus during the next week should be on portion size; you're not used to how much food your stomach can handle, so you will have to be careful. It's best to limit portions to 2 to 3 ounces during this time.

You can purée soft meats, fruits, cooked veggies, eggs, legumes, low-fat dairy, low-fat soups, and low-fiber cooked cereal. Just keep in mind that there should be no solid pieces in it at all—aim for a smooth paste. Also, don't neglect your hydration. You still have to drink water, as well as protein shakes during week three.

Some tips to get through this week:

- If you experience any discomfort while eating, make sure you're not eating too fast or taking bites that are too large.
- If you're not hungry, continue to drink your protein shakes. You must keep meeting your daily protein goals.
- Don't neglect your hydration. Remember, fluids first, then protein, and lastly, other foods.
- Try to eat ½ a cup of food for each meal.
- Continue to drink high-protein milk between each meal to up your protein intake.
- You can use water, milk, broth, or yogurt to thin foods to your desired consistency.

Your body is used to digesting puréed food now and is ready for food with more substance. As you introduce different types of softer protein into your diet, you can start to drink fewer protein shakes, but only if you're eating enough protein otherwise.

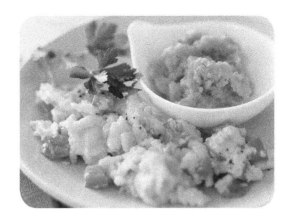

For food to be classified as 'soft,' it has to be tender enough for you to easily cut through it with a fork. Don't overwhelm your body by eating various types of soft foods in one meal—stick to adding one or two types of food at a time. Lean ground beef or poultry, soft and flaky fish, eggs, cottage cheese, soft cheese, yogurt, cooked vegetables, and canned fruits are good options to include on your menu in weeks six and seven.

Portions will vary, but you can aim for ½ cup of food per meal. Always adjust the nutritional information based on what you consumed to make sure you don't miss your protein target of 2.11 and 2.82 ounces per day. Again, don't forget to stay hydrated!

Some helpful tips for weeks four, five, and six:

- If you are experiencing discomfort after adding soft food, try eating something with more moisture.
- Set alarms to remind you to eat if you discover that you lack an appetite.
- Only introduce one or two new foods at a time.

Congratulations! You made it. You have completed the transition diet and can now add a variety of textures back into your diet. This doesn't mean you should forget to focus on portion size and making sure you're eating enough protein! These two aspects will continue with you throughout your life. Also, stay away from high-fat and high-carb foods.

As weeks four, five, and six, only introduced one or two new foods at a time, be mindful that some foods may cause some discomfort.

Portions will vary, but you should be able to comfortably ingest ½ to one cup of food each meal. Continue to reach your target of 48 ounces of fluids and 2.11 ounces of protein daily.

Going forward, remember to:

- Eat three meals with two snacks a day.
- Drink high-protein milk between meals to meet your protein target until you are able to eat enough protein.
- If you feel ill after introducing more solids, go back to following the soft food diet of weeks six and seven.
- Don't forget to drink water to keep yourself hydrated.

Dealing with Social Occasions

Humans like to gather around a table, enjoy some good food and a glass of wine. There's nothing wrong with your innate need to be social, but for someone who underwent weight-loss surgery, it can be a source of anxiety. There are certain limitations you have to consider when going out, but you should let it hold you back.

Dining Out

With some planning and quick thinking, you can join your friends at any restaurant and order with ease.

- Check the menu ahead of time. You can check the website, or if you know where the restaurant is, head in for a quick coffee and look over what you can order beforehand.
- There's no rule stopping you from ordering an appetizer or side-dish as an entrée.
- Do not be adventurous when eating out. Choose foods you know work well with your stomach.
- Remember the basics: no deep-fried foods, carbs, high-fat food, sweet carbonated drinks, or desserts.
- Divide your plate into two. You can eat the leftovers the next day.

During the Holidays

Holidays are full of temptation—food and alcohol at every turn. This combined with the excitement of spending time with family and friends may be enough to cause some missteps. Here are some tips on how to deal with parties and celebrations after you've had bariatric surgery.

- Eat a meal or snack that is high in protein before the party.
- Don't sit close to any appetizers or the buffet tables. You don't want to fall into the "it's there, so let me take one bite" trap.
- If you're asked to bring a side dish, make one that you'll be able to eat.
- Always choose a small portion of protein and vegetables from the menu or at a buffet.
- If you don't want to drink alcohol, but you're afraid everyone will make a fuss, fill a cocktail glass with water, and add some juice and a lemon wedge. Voilà! A sleeve-friendly mocktail.

FAQs

Vertical gastric sleeve surgery is such a life-changing surgery. I'm sure you have even more questions whirling around in your head than the ones I answered in this cookbook. Don't worry. I have a good idea of what you may want to know based on the questions I asked when I first learned about VGS and bariatric surgery in general.

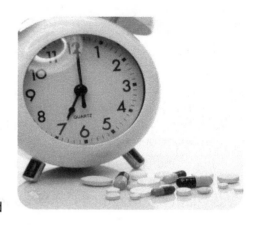

1. Can doctors refuse to do a VSG on me?

It's not so much that they'll refuse but recommend you get gastric bypass surgery instead in some instances. If you have difficulty swallowing (esophageal dysmotility) or if your food stays in your stomach too long (gastroparesis), gastric bypass is the better option. The same applies if you have severe GERD.

2. Do I need to change my diet before getting surgery?

Technically, you don't need to change your eating habits before VSG, but I suggest you try. If you start to make healthy changes to what you eat and create positive eating patterns beforehand, you'll have an easier time adjusting to the bariatric diet post-op. It is overwhelming to implement all the changes at once—counting protein, drinking more water, giving up fast food, remembering your multivitamin daily, all while recovering from surgery. Establishing some of these habits weeks or months before the operation will make the adjustment process so much more comfortable.

However, your doctor may place you on a pre-operative program to help you lose weight before surgery. This is to decrease belly fat and reduce the liver size, which will make the operation safer for you.

3. How is it possible to pull such a large part of the stomach through such a small incision?

The stomach can stretch significantly—holding up to 128 ounces of food when fully expanded. During the VSG, a tube will remove all the gas and liquids from the stomach. This decompresses the stomach, making it possible to remove up to 80%. The fact that the incision is 1.11 inches at most means you will experience a lot less pain after surgery.

4. Will I keep the weight off after surgery?

The short answer is yes; research shows sustained weight loss after VSG. However, as I mentioned earlier in the book, bariatric surgery is not magic— you will need to do your part to ensure and maintain success.

5. Can VSG cause heartburn?

The jury is out on this one as some patients report increased Gastroesophageal Reflux Disease (GERD), while others describe a decrease. It seems if the surgeon does not remove the upper part of the stomach (fundus), GERD is more prevalent in patients. This is something you can discuss with your doctor to determine if they pay extra attention to removing the fundus.

But don't worry, if you happen to be one of the people who get GERD as a side-effect, it can easily be managed with antacid medication and diet changes.

6. I haven't met my protein goal for the day. What can I eat to boost my protein intake?

Don't worry too much if you don't always hit your protein targets—if you eat enough protein 80 percent of the time, you'll be fine. To up your protein for the day, choose something that doesn't take a lot of time to prepare. Low-fat cottage cheese, Greek yogurt, eggs, and lunch meat are good options, but you can also drink a protein shake if you're not in the mood to eat anything. You can eat a high-protein breakfast the next day to make up for the shortfall you had the day before.

7. What protein powders are the best?

I think the protein and supplement aisle is probably the most overwhelming section of any grocery store. There are so many products—each claiming to be better than the other. I suggest going for whey protein isolate. Not only is it easy for the body to absorb, but it also contains high amounts of essential amino acids. If you're looking for a vegetarian or vegan option, you can try soy protein isolate. It's best to go for the unflavored kind since they are low in calories and free from artificial ingredients. If you have no other option than choosing a flavored protein powder, always select the sugar-free kind.

8. I am always so full after eating my protein that there's no room for vegetables and fruits. This can't be healthy?

I know that eating only protein for weeks may not seem like the healthiest thing to do, but keep in mind that it is only temporary. While your body is getting used to a smaller stomach and the subsequent digestion changes, you will drink a multivitamin that will make up for any nutrients you'll miss out on during this time. As you move from liquids to purée, and finally to regular eating patterns, your stomach will adjust, and you will have space for food other than protein.

9. There is so much conflicting information about carbohydrates. Am I allowed to eat carbs after VSG?

Your stomach will struggle to digest carbs for a few months after your surgery. This is why it is best to limit your carb intake. Another reason why most doctors suggest you cut carbs out of your diet is to help you lose weight. Carbohydrates are high in calories and will cause your weight loss to stall if eaten in excess. It also doesn't contain nearly the amount of vitamins and minerals fruits and veggies do. Considering that your stomach can only take so much, it is best to prioritize foods that will meet your nutritional needs.

10. How do I keep on track if I don't have support from my spouse?

It is difficult when the people in your household continue to eat junk food while you have to stick to the bariatric diet. The first thing you can do is communicate with your loved ones and let them know what you need. If they're not sure what your goals are and how you plan to reach them, you can't expect them to be considerate. However, here are some tips you can try when your family isn't willing to make a lifestyle change with you.

- Ask your family only to keep treats in the house that you can resist.
- Take up an activity that will keep your mind occupied or distract you when the Oreos in the cupboard is calling your name. Go for a walk, read, or call a support buddy—do anything you can to find an outlet that isn't eating.
- Keep healthy snacks or quick meals on hand for you and your family. If there is food in the house, you minimize the chances of a family member getting take-out because they're too hungry or tired to cook.

Lastly, if you're unlucky and your family doesn't care about your health journey, put all the unhealthy food in a cupboard with a lock and give only them keys. You'll still have to watch them eat these foods, but at least you won't have direct access to it when a craving strike.

Chapter 4

Full Liquid Diet

44   Almond and Cherry Shake

44   Lush Pumpkin Smoothie

45   Beef Bone Broth

45   Super Skim Milk

46   Chocolate and Peanut Smoothie

46   Coffee Protein Shake

48   Creamy Banana Shake

48   Strawberry Crème Shake

49   Chicken Bone and Vegetable Broth

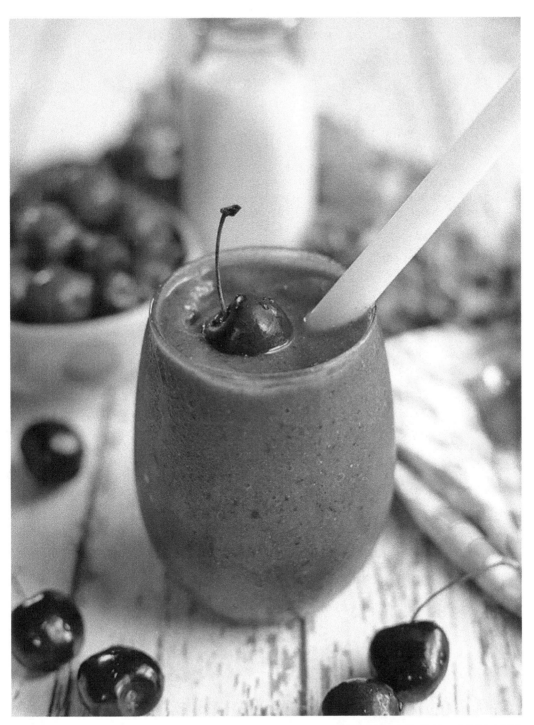

Almond and Cherry Shake

Prep time: 5 minutes | Cook time: 2 minutes | Serves: 2

- 1 (5.3-ounce / 150-g) cup low-fat black cherry yogurt
- ½ cup water
- ½ cup low-fat milk
- ¼ cup frozen pitted cherries
- ¼ cup vanilla protein powder
- ½ teaspoon almond extract

1. In a blender, blend on high speed to combine the yogurt, water, milk, cherries, protein powder, and almond extract for 2 to 3 minutes, until the shake is smooth and the protein powder is well dissolved.
2. Pour the shake into a glass and serve. Refrigerate any shake you don't drink.

Per Serving (1 cup)

calories: 158 | total carbs: 16.0g | protein: 20.0g | total fat: 1.0g | sugar: 12.0g
fiber: 0g | sodium: 89mg

Lush Pumpkin Smoothie

Prep time: 5 minutes | Cook time: 2 minutes | Serves: 2

- 1 cup low-fat milk
- ½ cup pumpkin purée
- ½ cup low-fat cottage cheese
- ¼ cup vanilla protein powder
- 1 teaspoon pumpkin pie spice
- 1 teaspoon vanilla extract

1. In a blender, blend on high speed to combine the milk, pumpkin purée, cottage cheese, protein powder, pumpkin pie spice, and vanilla for 2 to 3 minutes, until the smoothie is smooth and the powder is well dissolved.
2. Pour the smoothie into a glass and serve. Refrigerate any smoothie you don't drink.

Per Serving (1 cup)

calories: 196 | total carbs: 17.0g | protein: 25.0g | total fat: 2.0g | sugar: 6.0g
fiber: 3.0g | sodium: 392mg

Beef Bone Broth

Prep time: 1 hour | Cook time: 12+ hours | Makes: 12 cups

- 2 pounds (907 g) beef bones
- 1 gallon water
- 2 tablespoons apple cider vinegar
- 1 onion, roughly chopped
- 2 large carrots, roughly chopped
- 2 celery stalks, roughly chopped
- 1 tablespoon salt
- 1 teaspoon peppercorns
- 1 bunch fresh parsley
- 2 garlic cloves

1. Preheat the oven to 350°F (180°C).
2. Put the bones on a baking sheet and roast in the oven for 30 minutes. Flip the bones halfway through.
3. Transfer the bones to a stock pot, add the water and vinegar, and let sit for 30 minutes.
4. Add the onions, carrots, and celery, and bring to a boil.
5. Transfer to a slow cooker, and add the salt and peppercorns. Cook on low for 12 to 24 hours, using a spoon to periodically remove any impurities that float to the surface.
6. During the last 30 minutes of cooking, add the parsley and garlic.
7. Remove from the heat and let cool. Strain with a fine metal strainer.
8. Transfer to air-tight jars. Store in the refrigerator for up to 5 days or in the freezer for up to 3 months. For easy use in recipes, freeze in ice cube trays and then transfer to a large freezer bag.

`Per Serving`
calories: 69 | total carbs: 1.0g | protein: 6.0g | total fat: 4.0g | sugar: 19.0g
fiber: 1.0g | sodium: 263mg

Super Skim Milk

Prep time: 5 minutes | Cook time: 5 minutes | Serves: 4

- 4 cups skim milk
- 1 cup nonfat dry milk powder

1. In a deep bowl or a blender, beat the milk and milk powder slowly with a beater or blend on high speed to mix for about 5 minutes, until the powder is well dissolved.
2. Serve immediately. Or refrigerate the milk for up to a week.

`Per Serving`
calories: 144 | total carbs: 21.0g | protein: 14.0g | total fat: 0g | sugar: 21.0g
fiber: 0g | sodium: 218mg

Chocolate and Peanut Smoothie

Prep time: 5 minutes | Cook time: 3 minutes | Serves: 2

- 1 cup low-fat milk
- ½ cup low-fat plain Greek yogurt
- ¼ cup vanilla protein powder
- 2 tablespoons powdered peanut butter
- 2 tablespoons cocoa powder

1. In a blender, blend on high speed to combine the milk, yogurt, protein powder, powdered peanut butter, and cocoa powder for 3 to 4 minutes, until the powders are well dissolved and no longer visible.
2. Pour the smoothie into a glass and serve. Refrigerate any smoothie you don't drink.

Per Serving

calories: 185 | total carbs: 17.0g | protein: 24.0g | total fat: 3.0g | sugar: 10.0g fiber: 3.0g | sodium: 173mg

Coffee Protein Shake

Prep time: 5 minutes | Cook time: 3 minutes | Serves: 2

- 1 cup decaffeinated coffee, brewed and chilled
- 1 cup low-fat milk
- ¼ cup vanilla protein powder
- ½ teaspoon cinnamon
- ½ cup ice

1. In a blender, pour the coffee and milk, then add the protein powder, cinnamon, and ice. Blend on high speed, about 3 to 4 minutes, until the shake is smooth and the protein powder is well dissolved.
2. Pour the shake into a glass and serve. Refrigerate any shake you don't drink.

Per Serving

calories: 102 | total carbs: 8.0g | protein: 14.0g | total fat: 0g | sugar: 6.0g fiber: 0g | sodium: 155mg

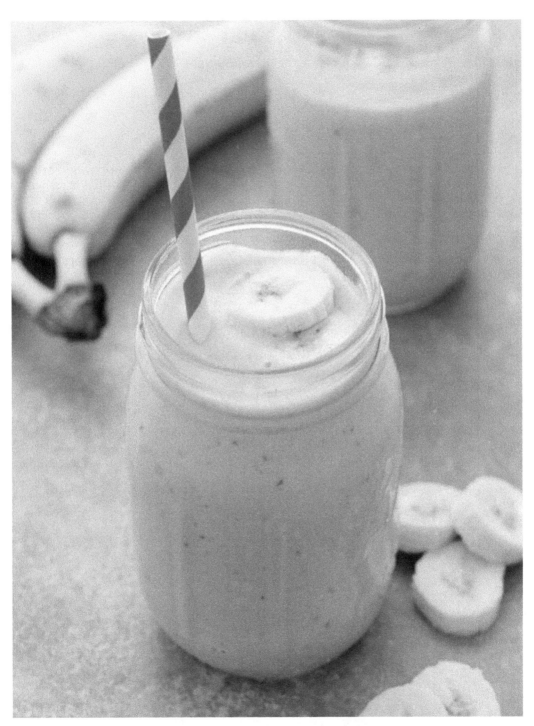

Creamy Banana Shake

Prep time: 5 minutes | Cook time: 2 minutes | Serves: 2

- 1½ cups low-fat milk
- ¼ cup plain Greek yogurt
- 1 small banana
- 1 teaspoon vanilla extract
- ¼ cup vanilla protein powder
- 1 tablespoon sugar-free banana pudding mix

1. In a blender, combine the milk, yogurt, banana, vanilla, protein powder, and pudding mix. Blend on high for 2 to 3 minutes, until the powder has dissolved and the mixture is smooth.
2. Pour the shake into a glass and serve. Refrigerate any shake you don't drink.

Per Serving

calories: 226 | total carbs: 30.0g | protein: 17.0g | total fat: 4.0g | sugar: 19.0g fiber: 1.0g | sodium: 263mg

Strawberry Crème Shake

Prep time: 5 minutes | Cook time: 2 minutes | Serves: 2

- 1 cup low-fat milk
- 1 cup fresh strawberries
- ½ cup plain Greek yogurt
- ¼ cup vanilla protein powder
- ½ teaspoon vanilla extract

1. In a blender, blend on high speed to combine the milk, strawberries, yogurt, protein powder, and vanilla for 2 to 3 minutes, until the shake is smooth and the protein powder is well dissolved.
2. Pour the shake into a glass and serve. Refrigerate any shake you don't drink.

Per Serving

calories: 145 | total carbs: 15.0g | protein: 15.0g | total fat: 2.0g | sugar: 6.0g fiber: 1.0g | sodium: 92mg

Chicken Bone and Vegetable Broth

Prep time: 5 minutes | Cook time: 5 to 8 hours | Makes: 8 cups

- 2 cups diced celery
- 1 medium yellow onion, sliced
- 4 large carrots, peeled and chopped
- 1 (5- to 7-pound / 2.3- to 3.2-kg) whole chicken
- 12 to 16 cups water
- 1 teaspoon salt
- 2 bay leaves
- Nonstick cooking spray

1. Preheat the oven to 400°F (205ºC). Coat a shallow roasting pan with cooking spray.
2. Arrange the celery, onion, and carrot in the roasting pan. Put the whole raw chicken in the pan. Roast for 90 minutes or more (about 20 minutes per pound of chicken), until a thermometer inserted in the thigh reads 165°F (74ºC) and the juices run clear.
3. Remove the pan from the oven and remove the meat from carcass, setting aside for other recipes.
4. Put the carcass and vegetables in a large pot. Add enough water to the pot to cover the carcass and vegetables completely. Add the salt and bay leaves to the pot and bring to a rolling boil.
5. Simmer over medium heat for at least 4 hours, or longer for increased flavor. Stir a few times each hour.
6. Use a strainer spoon to remove the bones and vegetables from the pot. Serve the broth warm.

Per Serving (2 cups broth)
calories: 138 | total carbs: 1.0g | protein: 15.0g | total fat: 2.0g | sugar: 0g
fiber: 0g | sodium: 400mg

Chapter 5

Puréed Foods

52	Avocado Milk Whip
52	Broccoli Purée
53	Banana and Kale Smoothie
53	Easy Chocolate and Orange Pudding
54	Matcha Mango Smoothie
54	Ricotta Peach Fluff
54	Blueberry and Spinach Smoothie
56	Simple Applesauce
56	Split Pea and Carrot Soup
57	Beef Purée
58	Herbed Chicken Purée

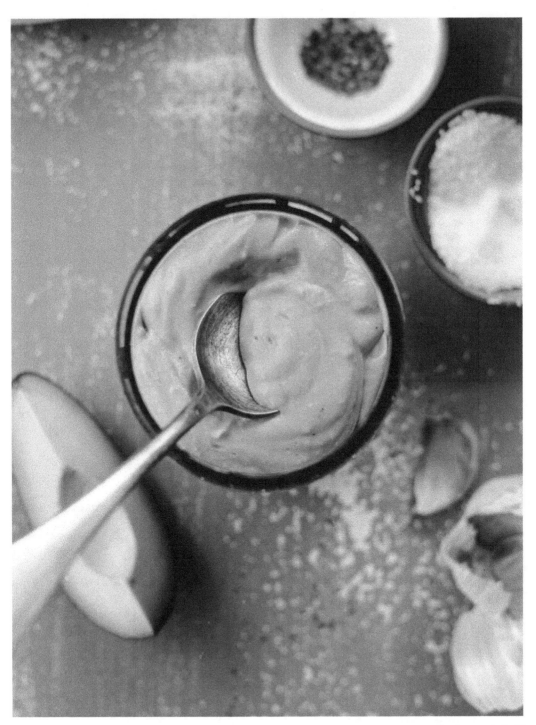

Avocado Milk Whip

Prep time: 10 minutes | Cook time: 0 minutes | Serves: 2

- 1 avocado, peeled, pitted, diced
- 1 cup skim milk
- ½ cup non-fat cottage cheese
- ¼ cup fresh cilantro leaves, stems

- removed
- ½ teaspoon lime juice
- ¼ teaspoon garlic powder
- Chili powder, for garnish

1. Put all ingredients in a blender and pulse until smooth.
2. Divide the whip between two bowls and sprinkle with a dash of chili powder to serve.

Per Serving

calories: 317 | total carbs: 26.6g | protein: 11.5g | total fat: 20.0g | sugar: 17.7g
fiber: 6.8g | sodium: 241mg

Broccoli Purée

Prep time: 30 minutes | Cook time: 10 minutes | Serves: 6

- 1 pound(454 g) fresh broccoli, cut into florets
- ½ cup water
- ½ teaspoon salt, plus more to taste
- 1 teaspoon butter

- 1 teaspoon lemon juice
- ½ teaspoon onion powder
- Freshly ground black pepper, to taste

1. Mix the broccoli florets, water and ½ teaspoon salt in a medium saucepan and bring to a simmer. Reduce heat, cover the pan and simmer until the broccoli is tender, 5 to 10 minutes.
2. Drain the broccoli, reserving the cooking water. Add the butter, lemon juice and onion powder, season with salt and pepper and let cool.
3. Put about 1 cup broccoli florets and ¼ cup cooking water in a food processor and pulse until smooth. Repeat with remaining broccoli.
4. Serve immediately.

Per Serving

calories: 28 | total carbs: 4.3g | protein: 2.4g | total fat: 0.9g | sugar: 1.g
fiber: 2.3g | sodium: 212mg

Banana and Kale Smoothie

Prep time: 5 minutes | Cook time: 0 minutes | Serves: 2

- 2 cups unsweetened almond milk
- 2 cups kale, stemmed, leaves chopped
- 2 bananas, peeled
- 1 to 2 packets stevia, or to taste
- 1 teaspoon ground cinnamon
- 1 cup crushed ice

1. In a blender, combine the almond milk, kale, bananas, stevia, cinnamon, and ice. Blend until smooth.
2. Serve immediately.

Per Serving

calories: 181 | total carbs: 37.0g | protein: 4.0g | total fat: 4.0g | sugar: 15.0g
fiber: 6.0g | sodium: 210mg

Easy Chocolate and Orange Pudding

Prep time: 5 minutes | Cook time: 5 minutes | Serves: 4

- 1 package sugar-free instant chocolate pudding mix
- ¼ cup chocolate protein powder
- 2 cups low-fat milk
- 1 tablespoon cocoa powder
- 1 teaspoon orange extract

1. In a small bowl, whisk the pudding and protein powders together with the milk for 2 minutes.
2. Add the cocoa powder and orange extract, and mix for 3 more minutes before serving.

Per Serving

calories: 111 | total carbs: 15.0g | protein: 10.0g | total fat: 2.0g | sugar: 6.0g
fiber: 1.0g | sodium: 380mg

Matcha Mango Smoothie

Prep time: 5 minutes | Cook time: 0 minutes | Serves: 2

- 2 cups cubed mango
- 2 tablespoons matcha powder
- 2 teaspoons turmeric powder
- 2 cups almond milk
- 2 tablespoons honey
- 1 cup crushed ice

1. In a blender, combine the mango, matcha, turmeric, almond milk, honey, and ice. Blend until smooth.
2. Serve immediately.

Per Serving

calories: 285 | total carbs: 68.0g | protein: 4.0g | total fat: 3.0g | sugar: 63.0g
fiber: 6.0g | sodium: 94mg

Ricotta Peach Fluff

Prep time: 10 minutes | Cook time: 0 minutes | Serves: 1

- ¼ cup ricotta cheese
- 1 ripe peach, diced
- 2 tablespoons skim milk

1. Purée ricotta, diced peach and milk in a blender until smooth.
2. Serve immediately.

Per Serving

calories: 355| total carbs: 54.0g | protein: 17.9g | total fat: 8.7g | sugar: 50.0g
fiber: 2.0g | sodium: 183mg

Blueberry and Spinach Smoothie

Prep time: 5 minutes | Cook time: 2 minutes | Serves: 4

- 2 cups blueberries
- 3 cups chopped fresh spinach
- ½ cup chopped fresh coriander
- Juice of 1 lemon
- 1-inch fresh ginger, grated
- 2 cups water

1. Put all the ingredients in the blender, pulse for 2 minutes or until smooth.
2. Serve immediately.

Per Serving

calories: 121 | total carbs: 30.0g | protein: 1.6g | total fat: 0.6g | sugar: 26.6g
fiber: 2.6g | sodium: 25mg

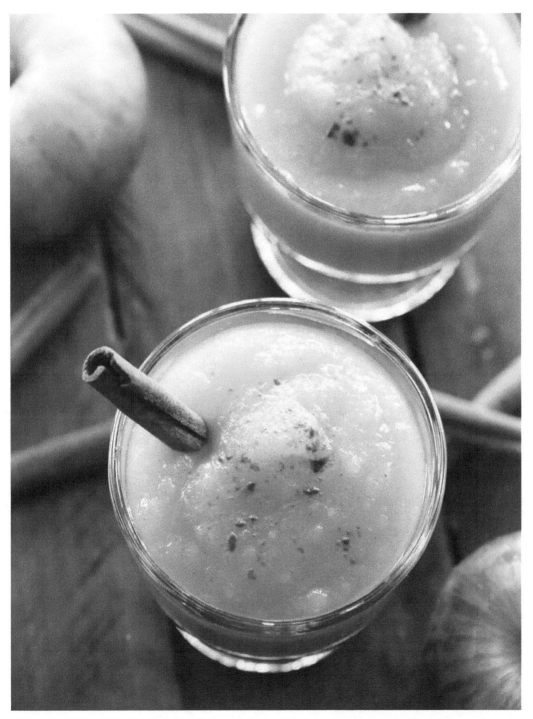

Simple Applesauce

Prep time: 10 minutes | Cook time: 15 minutes | Serves: 3

- 2 medium apples (peeled, cored, sliced)
- ¼ cup water, plus more if needed
- Dash cinnamon
- Dash nutmeg

1. Put all ingredients in a small saucepan and heat to a simmer. Cook, stirring frequently, until apples are very soft and falling apart, about 15 minutes.
2. Purée applesauce with an immersion blender until very smooth, adding more water if necessary.
3. Serve immediately or refrigerate applesauce until chilled through, about 1 hour, before serving.

Per Serving

calories: 63 | total carbs: 16.8g | protein: 0.3g | total fat: 0.2g | sugar: 12.6g fiber: 2.9g | sodium: 0mg

Split Pea and Carrot Soup

Prep time: 10 minutes | Cook time: 1 hour 10 minutes | Makes: 1 gallon

- 1 tablespoon extra-virgin olive oil
- 2 large carrots, chopped
- 1 medium onion, diced
- 2 garlic cloves, minced
- 4 cups chicken broth
- 2 cups water
- Salt, to taste
- Freshly ground black pepper, to taste
- 2 dried bay leaves
- 1 (16-ounce / 454-g) bag green split peas

1. In a large stock pot over medium heat, heat the oil.
2. Add the carrot, onion, and garlic. Sauté until soft, 5 to 7 minutes.
3. Add the broth, water, salt and pepper, bay leaves, and split peas. Stir well, and bring to a boil.
4. Reduce the heat to a simmer, cover, and let cook for 1 hour, or until the peas are soft.
5. Remove the bay leaves, and serve immediately.

Per Serving

calories: 92 | total carbs: 20.0g | protein: 8.0g | total fat: 1.0g | sugar: 2.0g fiber: 8.0g | sodium: 264mg

Beef Purée

Prep time: 30 minutes | Cook time: 4 to 10 hours | Serves: 4

- 1 pound (454 g) beef tenderloin steak
- 1 teaspoon olive oil
- 1 teaspoon soy sauce
- ½ teaspoon salt, plus more to taste
- ½ teaspoon garlic powder
- ½ teaspoon onion powder
- ½ teaspoon dried rosemary, crushed
- ½ teaspoon dried parsley
- ¼ teaspoon freshly ground black pepper, plus more to taste
- Beef stock, as needed

1. Pat the steak dry with paper towels and brush with olive oil and soy sauce. Mix salt, garlic powder, onion powder, rosemary, parsley and pepper and rub over steak. Cook the steak in a slow cooker until cooked through and the internal temperature reaches 145ºF (63ºC), 8 to 10 hours at the low setting or 4 to 5 hours at the high setting.
2. Remove the steak from slow cooker, reserving the cooking juices. Put the steak in a covered container and refrigerate until chilled through, about 2 hours.
3. Cut the chilled steak into 1-inch cubes. Put about 1 cup steak cubes in a food processor and pulse until fine and powdery. Add about ¼ cup reserved cooking juices plus stock as needed and process until smooth. Repeat with remaining steak cubes.
4. Season the puréed steak with salt and pepper and stir until thoroughly combined.
5. Serve immediately.

Per Serving

calories: 168 | total carbs: 1g | protein: 23.3g | total fat: 7.9g | sugar: 0.3g fiber: 0.2g | sodium: 410mg

Herbed Chicken Purée

Prep time: 30 minutes | Cook time: 30 minutes | Serves: 6

- 2 (8-ounce / 227-g) boneless skinless chicken breasts
- 2 bay leaves
- ¾ teaspoon salt, divided
- ¾ teaspoon ground sage
- ½ teaspoon ground thyme
- ¼ teaspoon ground marjoram
- ¼ teaspoon ground rosemary
- ¼ teaspoon freshly ground black pepper
- Dash of nutmeg

1. Put the chicken breasts, bay leaves, and 1/2 teaspoon in a medium saucepan, add enough cold water to cover and bring to a boil. Reduce the heat, cover and simmer gently until chicken is cooked through and the internal temperature reaches at least 165ºF (74ºC), 20 to 25 minutes.
2. Remove the chicken breasts from broth. Strain and reserve the broth. Put chicken in a covered container and refrigerate until chilled through, about 2 hours.
3. Cut the chilled chicken breasts into 1-inch cubes. Put about 1 cup chicken cubes in a food processor and pulse until fine and powdery. Add about ¼ cup reserved broth and process until smooth. Repeat with remaining chicken cubes.
4. Mix the sage, thyme, marjoram, rosemary, pepper and nutmeg with remaining salt, sprinkle over the puréed chicken and stir until thoroughly combined.
5. Serve immediately.

Per Serving
calories: 92 | total carbs: 0.2g | protein: 17.1g | total fat: 2g | sugar: 0g
fiber: 0.1g | sodium: 325mg

Chapter 6

Soft Foods

61   Hearty Gazpacho

61   Mango and Banana Porridge

62   Berries and Walnut Pops

62   Creamy Egg and Tuna Salad

63   Chia Protein Oatmeal

63   Creamy Cheese Berry Smoothies

65   Scrambled Eggs

65   Oat and Fruit Smoothie

66   Puréed Strawberries with Creamy Yogurt

66   Tomato Scrambled Egg with Bacon

67   Creamy Chicken and Vegetable Soup

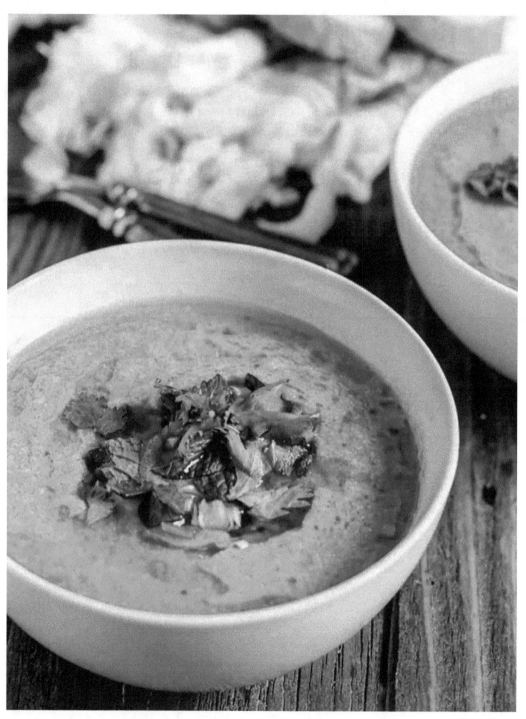

Hearty Gazpacho

Prep time: 15 minutes | Cook time: 6 minutes | Serves: 4

- 2 tablespoons vegetable oil
- 1 small red bell pepper, diced
- 1 small yellow onion, diced
- 2 garlic cloves, minced
- 4 large fresh ripe tomatoes, peeled, diced
- 1 small cucumber, peeled, diced
- 1 tablespoon lime juice
- 1 tablespoon balsamic vinegar
- 1 tablespoon chopped fresh basil leaves
- 1 teaspoon kosher salt, plus more to taste
- ½ teaspoon ground cumin
- Freshly ground black pepper, to taste

1. In a medium saucepan, heat the oil over medium heat and sauté the bell pepper and onion until softened, about 5 minutes, stirring occasionally. Add the garlic and sauté for 1 minute more, stirring constantly.
2. Remove the pan from heat and stir in tomatoes, cucumber, lime juice, vinegar, basil, salt and cumin and season with pepper.
3. Pour the mixture into a blender and pulse to desired consistency.
4. Refrigerate the soup for 2 hours. Serve chilled.

Per Serving

calories: 118 | total carbs: 12.3g | protein: 2.4g | total fat: 7.4g | sugar: 7.5g
fiber: 3.2g | sodium: 594mg

Mango and Banana Porridge

Prep time: 5 minutes | Cook time: 5 minutes | Serves: 2

- 1 cup coconut milk
- 3 tablespoons farina breakfast porridge mix
- ½ cup diced ripe mango
- 1 small banana, diced

1. Bring the coconut milk to a simmer in a small saucepan over medium heat. Whisk the farina into milk and stir until smooth.
2. Reduce the heat and simmer, uncovered, until the porridge is thickened, about 2 minutes. Remove the porridge from the heat and stir in the mango and banana to serve.

Per Serving

calories: 151 | total carbs: 25.3g | protein: 4.8g | total fat: 4.3g | sugar: 18.5g
fiber: 2.0g | sodium: 58mg

Berries and Walnut Pops

Prep time: 10 minutes | Cook time: 0 minutes | Serves: 6

- 2 cups plain unsweetened Greek yogurt
- 1 cup skim milk
- ½ cup chopped walnuts
- ½ cup chopped strawberries
- ½ cup blueberries
- ½ cup raspberries

1. Whisk the yogurt and milk in a bowl until smooth. Add the walnuts, strawberries, blueberries and raspberries and stir to combine, crushing berries as desired.
2. Spoon the mixture into 6 freezer pop molds, set handled lids in place and freeze until firm, about 4 hours. Pops can be stored in the freezer for about 2 weeks.
3. Serve chilled.

Per Serving

calories: 102 | total carbs: 10.5g | protein: 4.1g | total fat: 5.4g | sugar: 8.6g
fiber: 1.2g | sodium: 42mg

Creamy Egg and Tuna Salad

Prep time: 15 minutes | Cook time: 0 minutes | Serves: 2

- 2 tablespoons plain unsweetened Greek yogurt
- 1 tablespoon mayonnaise
- 1 tablespoon skim milk
- 1 teaspoon yellow mustard
- 1 hard boiled egg, peeled
- 1 teaspoon minced fresh chives
- ¼ teaspoon onion powder
- 1 (6-ounce / 170-g) can tuna in water, drained
- Salt and freshly ground black pepper, to taste

1. Mix the yogurt, mayonnaise, milk and mustard. Mash the egg with a fork and stir into the yogurt mixture with chives and onion powder.
2. Flake the tuna and break into small pieces with a fork. Add the tuna to yogurt mixture and season with salt and pepper.
3. Serve immediately.

Per Serving

calories: 225 | total carbs: 17.5g | protein: 24.2g | total fat: 6.2g | sugar: 16.8g
fiber: 0.2g | sodium: 380mg

Chia Protein Oatmeal

Prep time: 5 minutes | Cook time: 10 minutes | Serves: 1

- ½ cup skim milk
- ¼ teaspoon vanilla extract
- 1 cup water
- Salt, to taste
- 2 teaspoons chia seeds

- ½ cup old-fashioned oats
- 2 tablespoons vanilla-flavored low-carb whey or soy protein isolate powder
- 1 teaspoon sliced almonds, toasted

1. In a small saucepan over medium heat, mix the milk, vanilla extract, water, and salt. Bring the mixture to a boil, stirring occasionally.
2. Add the chia seeds to the saucepan, reduce heat and simmer until softened, 7 to 8 minutes, stirring occasionally.
3. Add the oats to pan and simmer for about 2 minutes, stirring constantly. Remove the oatmeal from heat, add the whey and stir until thoroughly combined.
4. Sprinkle the almonds over the oatmeal and serve.

Per Serving

calories: 237 | total carbs: 13.0g | protein: 33.0g | total fat: 0g | sugar: 6.0g fiber: 5.0g | sodium: 80mg

Creamy Cheese Berry Smoothies

Prep time: 10 minutes | Cook time: 0 minutes | Serves: 2

- 1 cup mixed berries
- 2 tablespoons cream cheese
- 2 cups skim milk

- ¼ teaspoon vanilla extract
- 8 to 10 ice cubes

1. Put all the ingredients in a blender and pulse until thoroughly blended and smooth.
2. Pour into 2 large glasses to serve.

Per Serving

calories: 182 | total carbs: 21.0g | protein: 10.0g | total fat: 5.0g | sugar: 17.0g fiber: 3.0g | sodium: 175mg

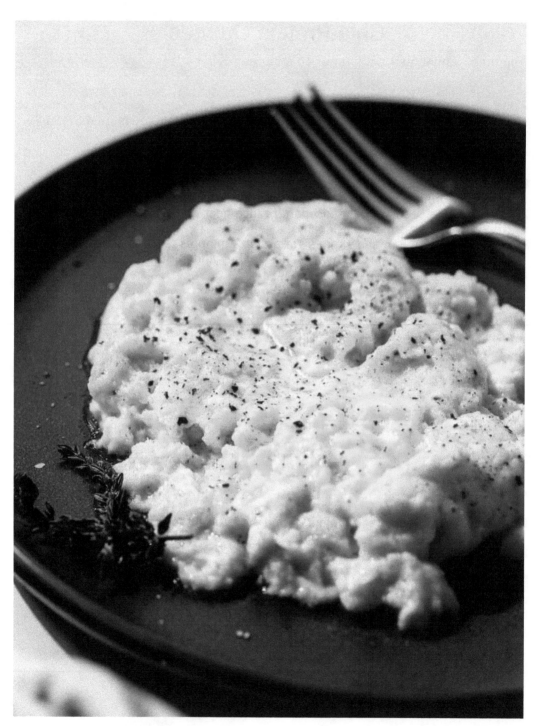

Scrambled Eggs

Prep time: 5 minutes | Cook time: 5 minutes | Serves: 2

- 2 eggs
- 1 tablespoon low-fat milk
- ½ teaspoon dried thyme
- Freshly ground black pepper, to taste
- Nonstick cooking spray

1. Set a small skillet over medium heat and coat the bottom of the skillet with cooking spray.
2. In a small bowl, beat the eggs lightly, then beat in the milk and thyme.
3. Add the egg mixture to the skillet, and turn down the heat to medium-low.
4. Stir the eggs gently and constantly with a spatula for 4 to 5 minutes, until they are fluffy and cooked thoroughly.
5. Season with black pepper and serve.

Per Serving

calories: 87 | total carbs: 1.0g | protein: 7.0g | total fat: 6.0g | sugar: 0g fiber: 0g | sodium: 83mg

Oat and Fruit Smoothie

Prep time: 10 minutes | Cook time: 0 minutes | Serves: 2

- ⅔ cup old-fashioned rolled oats
- ⅔ cup fat-free Greek yogurt
- 1 large banana, sliced and frozen
- ¼ cup plus 2 tablespoons coconut water, chilled
- Pinch of salt
- Vanilla extract, to taste
- 1 apple, cored and chopped
- 1 tablespoon flaked coconut
- 1 tablespoon mixed seeds and nuts

1. Purée the oats with the yogurt, banana, coconut water, salt and vanilla extract in a blender until smooth.
2. Pour the mixture into bowls and top with the apple, coconut, and mixed seeds and nuts to serve.

Per Serving

calories: 312 | total carbs: 54.7g | protein: 25.0g | total fat: 5.3g | sugar: 28.1g fiber: 9.5g | sodium: 211mg

Puréed Strawberries with Creamy Yogurt

Prep time: 10 minutes | Cook time: 7 minutes | Serves: 2

- 1 cup sliced strawberries
- 1 cup (8-ounce / 227-g) plain
- Greek yogurt
- 3 tablespoons heavy cream

1. Pulse the strawberries in a food processor until puréed. Set aside.
2. In a medium bowl, beat the yogurt and cream with an electric hand mixer until thickened and stiff peaks form, about 5 minutes.
3. Spoon the strawberries into two bowls, top with whipped yogurt and serve immediately.

Per Serving

calories: 175 | total carbs: 11.9g | protein: 5.2g | total fat: 12.5g | sugar: 9.9g
fiber: 1.4g | sodium: 66mg

Tomato Scrambled Egg with Bacon

Prep time: 5 minutes | Cook time: 14 minutes | Serves: 1

- 1 egg
- 1 teaspoon pesto
- 1 clove garlic, minced
- 2 cherry tomatoes, quartered
- 1 piece turkey bacon, crumbled
- 1 teaspoon Parmesan cheese, grated
- Cooking spray

1. Lightly whisk the egg in a mixing bowl. Add a dash of water and pesto. Whisk to combine well.
2. Spray a skillet with cooking spray and heat to medium-high.
3. Sauté the garlic for a minute or until fragrant. Stir in the bacon and cook for 4 minutes or until browned and crispy.
4. Remove the bacon and garlic from the skillet. Add the tomatoes to the skillet and sauté for 8 minutes or until liquid is almost gone.
5. Add the egg mixture to the skillet and sauté for a minute to scramble the eggs. Turn off the heat and stir in the bacon and garlic, and Parmesan cheese.
6. Serve immediately

Per Serving

calories: 211 | total carbs: 4.2g | protein: 12.8g | total fat: 15.9g | sugar: 1.6g
fiber: 0.5g | sodium: 340mg

Creamy Chicken and Vegetable Soup

Prep time: 30 minutes | Cook time: 50 minutes | Serves: 8

- 2 (8-ounce / 227-g) boneless skinless chicken breasts
- 6 cups water
- 1 (1-ounce / 28-g) onion, quartered
- 2 bay leaves
- 1 teaspoon garlic salt
- 2 cups chopped mixed vegetables
- (such as onions, carrots, celery, green beans or bell peppers)
- Salt and freshly ground black pepper, to taste
- 4 tablespoons butter
- 4 tablespoons flour
- 2 cups skim milk

1. Put the chicken breasts, water, onion, bay leaves and garlic salt in a large saucepan and bring to a boil. Reduce the heat, cover and simmer until chicken is cooked through, about 30 minutes.
2. Remove chicken breasts from the broth. Strain the broth, discarding the solids.
3. Add the mixed vegetables to the broth, season with salt and pepper and bring to a boil. Reduce the heat, cover and simmer until the vegetables are tender, about 20 minutes.
4. Meanwhile, cut the chicken into bite-size pieces and set aside. Melt the butter in a small nonstick skillet. Sprinkle the flour over butter and whisk until smooth. Add the milk to skillet in a thin stream, whisking constantly.
5. Bring the milk mixture to a simmer, whisking occasionally. Simmer for 2 minutes, whisking constantly.
6. Add the milk mixture to broth and whisk to combine. Add the chicken to soup and stir until heated through. Season the soup with salt and pepper and serve.

Per Serving
calories: 213 | total carbs: 18.4g | protein: 16.1g | total fat: 8.3g | sugar: 11.0g
fiber: 1.3g | sodium: 219mg

Chapter 7

Breakfast

70   Avocado and Egg Toast

70   Southwest Egg and Vegetable Scramble

71   Simple Cottage Pancakes

71   Mini Egg White Pizza

72   Yogurt and Mixed Berry Crumble

72   Spinach Quiche

74   Baked Oatmeal with Cherries and Apple

75   Butternut Squash and Cauliflower Hash Browns

76   Pumpkin and Zucchini Muffins

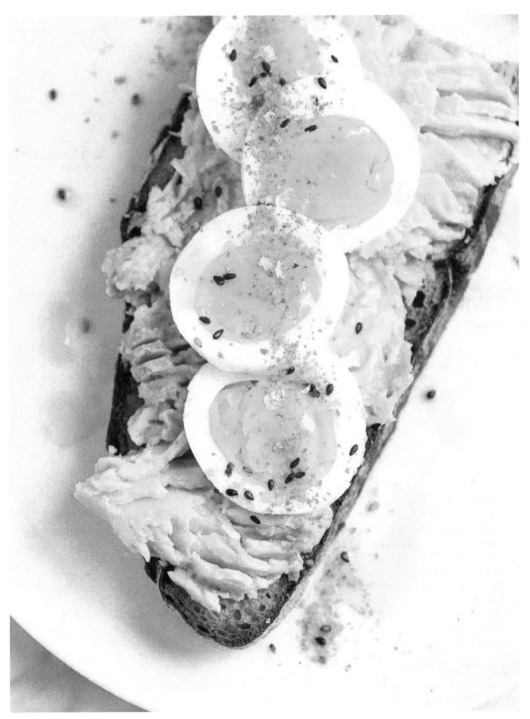

Avocado and Egg Toast

Prep time: 10 minutes | Cook time: 10 minutes | Makes: 2 toasts

- 4 eggs
- 1 medium avocado
- 4 slices sprouted whole-wheat bread,

toasted
- 1 teaspoon hot sauce
- Freshly ground black pepper, to taste

1. Bring a large pot of water to a rapid boil over high heat.
2. Carefully add the eggs to the boiling water using a spoon, and boil for 10 minutes.
3. Immediately transfer the eggs from the boiling water to a strainer, and run cold water over the eggs.
4. Once the eggs are cool enough to handle, peel them and slice lengthwise into fourths.
5. Mash the avocado with a fork in a small bowl and mix in the hot sauce.
6. Spread the avocado mash evenly across each toasted bread, then top with 4 egg slices and season with the black pepper.
7. Serve immediately.

Per Serving (1 toast)
calories: 191 | total carbs: 15.0g | protein: 10.0g | total fat: 10.0g | sugar: 1.0g
fiber: 5.0g | sodium: 214mg

Southwest Egg and Vegetable Scramble

Prep time: 5 minutes | Cook time: 10 minutes | Serves: 4

- 8 teaspoons extra-virgin olive oil
- 8 large eggs
- ½ cup diced red or yellow onion
- ½ cup diced bell pepper
- ½ cup canned diced tomatoes,

drained
- ¼ teaspoon salt
- Ground black pepper, to taste
- ½ cup sliced avocado

1. In a large skillet, heat the oil over medium-high heat.
2. In a medium bowl, beat the eggs well for about 1 minute. Set aside.
3. Add the onion and pepper to the skillet and cook, stirring frequently, for about 5 minutes, until the onion is translucent.
4. Add the beaten egg and cook for 1 to 2 minutes until the egg is cooked well, stirring frequently.
5. Add the diced tomato and cook for an additional 1 to 2 minutes. Remove from the heat.
6. Sprinkle the scramble with salt and pepper. Top the egg scramble with sliced avocado.
7. Serve immediately.

Per Serving (¾ to 1 cup)
calories: 266 | total carbs: 6.0g | protein: 14.0g | total fat: 21.0g | sugar: 2.0g
fiber: 2.0g | sodium: 292mg

Simple Cottage Pancakes

Prep time: 5 minutes | Cook time: 5 minutes | Makes: 4 pancakes

- 3 eggs
- 1 cup low-fat cottage cheese
- ⅓ cup whole-wheat pastry flour
- 1½ tablespoons coconut oil, melted
- Nonstick cooking spray

1. In large bowl, lightly whisk the eggs.
2. Whisk in the cottage cheese, flour, and coconut oil until combined.
3. Heat a large skillet over medium heat, and lightly coat with the cooking spray.
4. Pour ⅓ cup of the batter into the skillet for each pancake. Cook for 2 to 3 minutes, or until bubbles appear across the surface of each pancake. Flip the pancakes and cook for 1 to 2 more minutes, or until golden brown.
5. Serve immediately.

Per Serving (1 pancake)
calories: 182 | total carbs: 10.0g | protein: 12.0g | total fat: 10.0g | sugar: 1.0g
fiber: 3.0g | sodium: 68mg

Mini Egg White Pizza

Prep time: 5 minutes | Cook time: 5 minutes | Serves: 4

- 1 tablespoon extra-virgin olive oil
- 12 large egg whites (about 1½ cups egg whites)
- ½ teaspoon Italian seasoning
- ½ teaspoon garlic powder
- ¼ teaspoon salt
- ½ cup shredded Mozzarella cheese
- 1 cup sliced tomato (about 1 large tomato)

1. In a large skillet, heat the oil over medium heat.
2. In a large bowl, beat the egg whites with the Italian seasoning, garlic powder, and salt.
3. Pour the mixture into the skillet and cover with a lid. Cook for 1 to 2 minutes, or until egg whites start to bubble. Use a spatula to carefully lift at the edges to ensure the egg whites are not sticking to the skillet.
4. Remove the lid and sprinkle the Mozzarella cheese over the eggs. Put the tomato slices on top. Cover and heat for another 1 or 2 minutes until the cheese melts.
5. Carefully remove the egg white pizza from the pan. Divide into quarters and serve hot..

Per Serving (¾ cup)
calories: 180 | total carbs: 6.0g | protein: 19.0g | total fat: 11.0g | sugar: 3.0g
fiber: 1.0g | sodium: 486mg

Yogurt and Mixed Berry Crumble

Prep time: 5 minutes | Cook time: 5 minutes | Serves: 2

- 2 tablespoons almond flour
- ½ teaspoon ground cinnamon
- ¼ teaspoon stevia
- ½ tablespoon unsalted butter
- 2 tablespoons frozen or fresh diced strawberries
- 2 tablespoons frozen or fresh blueberries
- 1 cup nonfat plain Greek yogurt
- 1 teaspoon vanilla extract

1. In a small bowl, combine the almond flour, cinnamon, and stevia.
2. In a small skillet, combine the butter and almond flour mixture over medium heat. Cook for 1 to 2 minutes, stirring frequently as the butter melts. Once the moisture from the butter is absorbed and the mixture starts to crisp and clump a bit, remove the mixture from heat. Set the almond flour mixture aside in a separate bowl and carefully wipe out the skillet.
3. Put the strawberries and blueberries in the skillet and cook for 2 to 3 minutes, stirring frequently until softened. Remove from the heat.
4. In a small bowl, mix the yogurt with the vanilla extract. Layer the yogurt, fruit, and almond flour mixture in two serving bowls and enjoy.

Per Serving (¹⁄₃ cup)

calories: 147 | total carbs: 11.0g | protein: 14.0g | total fat: 7.0g | sugar: 8.0g
fiber: 2.0g | sodium: 44mg

Spinach Quiche

Prep time: 5 minutes | Cook time: 25 minutes | Serves: 4

- 1 cup chopped spinach
- 4 large eggs
- ½ cup shredded Cheddar cheese
- ¼ teaspoon salt
- Nonstick cooking spray

1. Preheat the oven to 350°F (180°C).
2. Line a muffin tin with 8 cupcake liners and spray each liner with nonstick cooking spray.
3. Fill the bottom of a medium saucepan with a couple inches of water and insert a steamer basket. Bring the water to a boil, then place the spinach in the steamer basket and cook for 3 minutes. Remove from the heat and drain well in a colander, pressing with the back of a spoon to remove the liquid.
4. In a medium mixing bowl, combine the spinach, eggs, Cheddar cheese, and salt. Pour the mixture evenly into the lined cups.
5. Bake for 15 to 20 minutes, or until a toothpick inserted in the middle of a quiche comes out clean. Serve warm.

Per Serving (2 egg quiches)

calories: 128 | total carbs: 1.0g | protein: 10.0g | total fat: 9.0g | sugar: 1.0g
fiber: 1.0g | sodium: 312mg

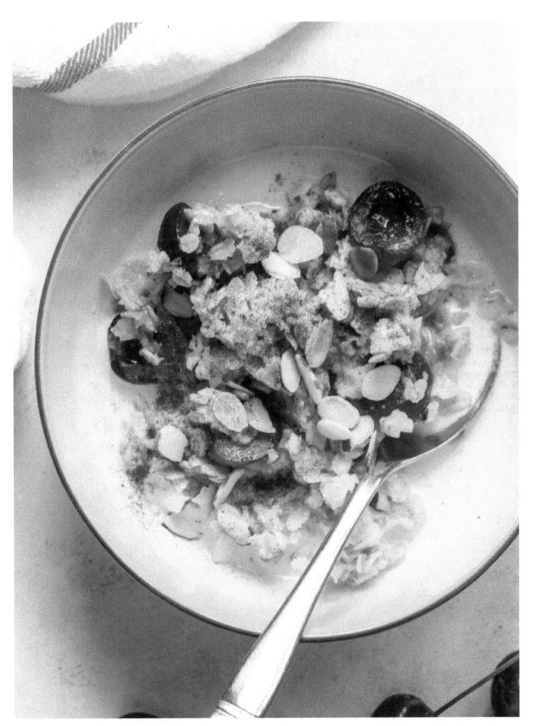

Baked Oatmeal with Cherries and Apple

Prep time: 10 minutes | Cook time: 45 minutes | Serves: 6

- 1 cup old-fashioned oats
- ½ teaspoon ground cinnamon
- ¾ teaspoon baking powder
- 1 tablespoon ground flaxseed
- 3 eggs
- 1 cup low-fat milk

- ½ cup low-fat plain Greek yogurt
- 1 teaspoon vanilla extract
- 1 teaspoon liquid stevia
- 1 cup fresh pitted cherries
- 1 apple, peeled, cored and chopped
- Nonstick cooking spray

1. Preheat the oven to 375°F (190ºC). Lightly coat a baking dish with cooking spray.
2. Mix together the oats, cinnamon, baking powder, and flaxseed in a medium bowl. In a separate large bowl, gently whisk the eggs, milk, yogurt, vanilla, and stevia.
3. Add the dry ingredients to the wet and stir to combine. Gently fold in the cherries and apples.
4. Bake in the preheated oven for 45 minutes or until the edges start to pull away from the side of the pan and the oatmeal gently bounces back when touched.
5. Serve immediately.

Per Serving (½ cup)
calories: 149 | total carbs: 21.0g | protein: 8.0g | total fat: 4.0g | sugar: 9.0g
fiber: 4.0g | sodium: 71mg

Butternut Squash and Cauliflower Hash Browns

Prep time: 10 minutes | Cook time: 50 minutes | Serves: 4

- 1 tablespoon extra-virgin olive oil
- 1 cup peeled and diced butternut squash
- 1 cup cauliflower rice
- ½ cup water
- ¼ teaspoon salt
- 2 large eggs
- ½ cup shredded Cheddar cheese
- ½ cup almond flour

1. Preheat the oven to 400°F (205ºC).
2. In a large skillet, heat the oil over medium heat. Add the diced butternut squash and cook for 10 to 12 minutes, stirring frequently.
3. Add the riced cauliflower, water, and salt to the skillet. Cook for 8 to 10 minutes and stir frequently until water is absorbed. Remove from the heat and cool for 5 to 7 minutes.
4. Take a large piece of cheesecloth and drape it open over a large mixing bowl. Then scoop the mixture into the center of the cheesecloth and bring all corners of the cloth together. Over top of the bowl, twist the cloth closed around the mixture and squeeze as much liquid out of the vegetable mixture as possible.
5. Remove the cheesecloth and place the drained mixture back into its original bowl. Add the eggs, Cheddar cheese, and almond flour and whisk to combine well.
6. Line a baking sheet with parchment paper. To form each patty, gather the mixture into 2 heaping tablespoons and space about 1 inch apart. Flatten each mound of mixture into a round patty shape.
7. Bake the hash browns in the oven for about 20 minutes or until golden brown and crispy.
8. Serve immediately.

Per Serving (2 hash browns)
calories: 197 | total carbs: 10.0g | protein: 11.0g | total fat: 14.0g | sugar: 2.0g
fiber: 4.0g | sodium: 278mg

Pumpkin and Zucchini Muffins

Prep time: 10 minutes | Cook time: 25 minutes | Makes: 2 dozen muffins

- 2 cups old-fashioned oats
- 1¾ cups whole-wheat pastry flour
- ¼ cup ground flaxseed
- 2 tablespoons baking powder
- 1 teaspoon baking soda
- 1 teaspoon ground cinnamon
- ¼ teaspoon ground nutmeg
- ¼ teaspoon ground ginger
- ¼ teaspoon ground allspice
- 2 cups shredded zucchini
- 1 cup fresh pumpkin purée
- 1 cup low-fat milk
- 4 eggs, lightly beaten
- ¼ cup unsweetened applesauce
- 1 teaspoon liquid stevia
- ½ cup chopped walnuts
- Nonstick cooking spray

1. Preheat the oven to 375°F (190ºC). Prepare two muffin tins by coating the cups with the cooking spray.
2. In large bowl, mix together the oats, flour, flaxseed, baking powder, baking soda, cinnamon, nutmeg, ginger, and allspice.
3. In a separate medium bowl mix together the zucchini, pumpkin, milk, eggs, applesauce, and stevia.
4. Add the wet ingredients to the dry and stir to combine. Gently stir in the walnuts.
5. Fill the cups of the muffin tins about half full with the batter.
6. Bake until the muffins are done, when a toothpick inserted in the center comes out clean, about 25 minutes.
7. Let the muffins cool for 5 minutes before removing them from the tins. Put on a baking rack to cool before serving.
8. Wrap leftover muffins in plastic wrap and freeze. Reheat the frozen muffins in the microwave for about 20 seconds.

Per Serving (1 muffin)

calories: 128 | total carbs: 18.0g | protein: 5.0g | total fat: 5.0g | sugar: 1.0g
fiber: 3.0g | sodium: 86mg

Chapter 8

Sides and Snacks

79   Caprese Skewers

79   Deviled Eggs

80   Adobo Black Bean Hummus

80   Radish Chips

81   Cauliflower Mash

81   Garden Vegetable Roast

83   Spinach Dip

83   Cucumber and Tomato Salad

84   Vegetable Deli Turkey Rolls

84   Zucchini Fries

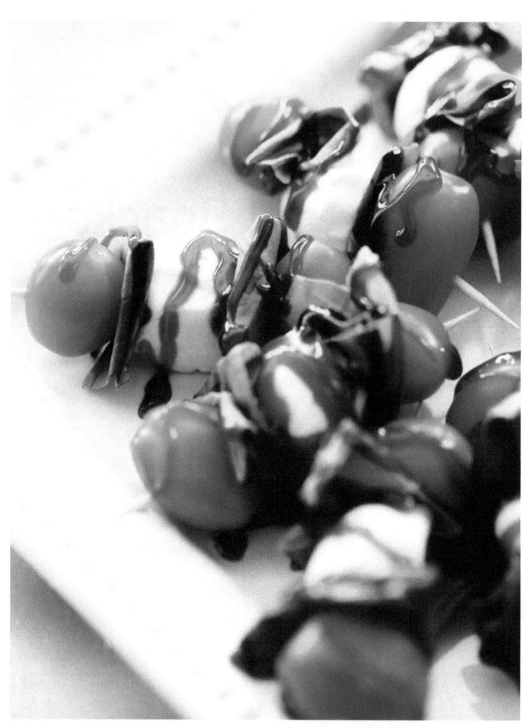

Caprese Skewers

Prep time: 10 minutes | Cook time: 15 minutes | Serves: 12

For the Bites:
- 24 cherry tomatoes
- 12 Mozzarella balls
- 12 fresh basil leaves

For the Balsamic Glaze:
- ½ cup balsamic vinegar
- 2 tablespoons extra-virgin olive oil
- 1 garlic clove, minced
- 1 teaspoon Italian seasoning

Special Equipment:
- 12 toothpicks, soaked in water for at least 30 minutes

To make the bites
1. Using 12 toothpicks, assemble each with 1 cherry tomato, 1 Mozzarella ball, 1 basil leaf, and another tomato. Put on a serving platter.

To make the glaze
2. In a small saucepan, bring the balsamic to a simmer, then simmer for 15 minutes, or until syrupy. Set aside to cool and thicken.
3. In a small bowl, whisk the olive oil, garlic, Italian seasoning, and cooled vinegar.
4. Drizzle the olive oil and balsamic glaze over the skewers. Serve immediately.

Per Serving

calories: 39 | total carbs: 3.0g | protein: 1.0g | total fat: 3.0g | sugar: 0g
fiber: 0g | sodium: 11mg

Deviled Eggs

Prep time: 10 minutes | Cook time: 0 minutes | Serves: 6

- 6 large hard-boiled eggs
- 2 tablespoons plain Greek yogurt
- ¼ teaspoon spicy mustard
- ⅛ teaspoon salt
- ½ teaspoon Taco seasoning

1. Peel the eggs, and halve them lengthwise.
2. Remove the yolks, and transfer them to a small bowl, setting the whites aside.
3. Add the yogurt, spicy mustard, salt, and taco seasoning to the bowl with the yolks, and mash everything together.
4. Spoon the mixture into the egg white halves, and serve.

Per Serving

calories: 83 | total carbs: 1.0g | protein: 7.0g | total fat: 5.0g | sugar: 1.0g
fiber: 0g | sodium: 129mg

Adobo Black Bean Hummus

Prep time: 5 minutes | Cook time: 5 minutes | Makes: 1½ cups

- 1 (15.5-ounce / 439-g) can black beans, drained and rinsed
- Juice of 1 lime
- 1 chipotle pepper in adobo sauce
- 1 teaspoon adobo sauce
- 1 teaspoon minced garlic
- 2 teaspoons ground cumin
- 2 tablespoons extra-virgin olive oil
- ¼ cup chopped fresh cilantro

1. In a food processor or blender, purée the black beans, lime juice, chipotle pepper, adobo sauce, garlic, cumin, olive oil, and cilantro on high until very smooth, 2 to 3 minutes.
2. Serve immediately.

Per Serving (2 tablespoons)
calories: 52 | total carbs: 6.0g | protein: 2.0g | total fat: 2.0g | sugar: 0g
fiber: 2.0g | sodium: 26mg

Radish Chips

Prep time: 5 minutes | Cook time: 35 minutes | Makes: 1 cup

- 1 cup thinly sliced radishes (2 bunches radishes)
- 1 tablespoon extra-virgin olive oil
- 3 tablespoons nutritional yeast
- flakes
- ¼ teaspoon salt
- Dash freshly ground black pepper (optional)

1. Preheat the oven to 375°F (190ºC). Line a baking sheet with parchment paper.
2. Put the radishes into a small bowl and toss in the oil.
3. In a small cup, mix the nutritional yeast, salt, and pepper (if using).
4. Put the oil-coated radish slices onto the prepared baking sheet in a single layer and sprinkle the nutritional yeast mixture lightly onto each slice.
5. Bake in the oven for about 15 minutes, then flip the chips and bake for another 15 minutes. Remove crispy chips, then continue to bake any remaining chips for a few minutes more at a time, until crispy and golden brown.
6. Serve immediately.

Per Serving (½ cup chips)
calories: 99 | total carbs: 4.0g | protein: 5.0g | total fat: 7.0g | sugar: 0g
fiber: 2.0g | sodium: 313mg

Cauliflower Mash

Prep time: 10 minutes | Cook time: 5 minutes | Makes: 3 cups

- 1 large head cauliflower, break into florets
- ¼ cup water
- ⅓ cup low-fat buttermilk
- 1 tablespoon minced garlic
- 1 tablespoon extra-virgin olive oil

1. Put the cauliflower florets in a large microwave-safe bowl with the water. Cover and microwave for about 5 minutes, or until the cauliflower is soft. Drain the water from the bowl.
2. In a blender or food processor, purée the buttermilk, cauliflower, garlic, and olive oil on medium speed until the cauliflower is smooth and creamy.
3. Serve immediately.

Per Serving (½ cup)
calories: 62 | total carbs: 8.0g | protein: 3.0g | total fat: 2.0g | sugar: 3.0g
fiber: 3.0g | sodium: 54mg

Garden Vegetable Roast

Prep time: 5 minutes | Cook time: 30 minutes | Serves: 6

- 1 small zucchini, sliced into rounds
- 1 medium bell pepper, cut into strips
- 1 small onion, halved then sliced
- 1 pint grape tomatoes
- 2 tablespoons extra-virgin olive oil
- Salt, to taste
- Freshly ground black pepper, to taste

1. Preheat the oven to 400°F (205ºC).
2. Using 1 or 2 large baking sheets, arrange the vegetables so they are lying flat, lightly touching each other.
3. Evenly pour the olive oil over the vegetables, and gently toss to coat, using either a spoon or your hands. Add salt and pepper to taste.
4. Roast in the preheated oven for 20 to 30 minutes, or until soft and lightly charred, stirring halfway through, and serve.

Per Serving
calories: 75 | total carbs: 8.0g | protein: 0g | total fat: 5.0g | sugar: 4.0g
fiber: 1.0g | sodium: 2mg

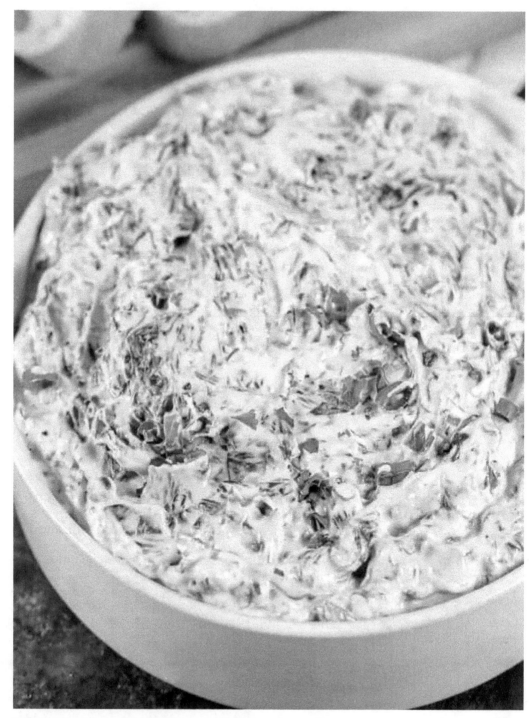

Spinach Dip

Prep time: 10 minutes | Cook time: 0 minutes | Serves: 12

- 1 cup plain nonfat Greek yogurt
- 4 ounces (113 g) Neufchâtel cheese
- ½ cup olive oil-based mayonnaise
- 2 teaspoons minced garlic
- 1½ teaspoons onion powder
- 1 teaspoon smoked paprika
- ¾ teaspoon freshly ground black pepper
- ¼ teaspoon red pepper flakes
- 2 teaspoons Worcestershire sauce
- 1 (8-ounce / 227-g) can water chestnuts, drained and finely chopped
- ½ cup chopped scallions
- 1 (10-ounce / 283-g) package frozen chopped spinach, thawed and squeezed of excess moisture

1. In a large bowl, use a hand mixer on low speed to mix the yogurt, Neufchâtel cheese, mayonnaise, garlic, onion powder, paprika, black pepper, red pepper flakes, and Worcestershire sauce.
2. Add the water chestnuts, scallions, and spinach and stir by hand until well combined.
3. Cover and refrigerate for at least 2 hours before serving.

Per Serving (¼ cup)
calories: 71 | total carbs: 5.0g | protein: 3.0g | total fat: 4.0g | sugar: 2.0g
fiber: 1.0g | sodium: 131mg

Cucumber and Tomato Salad

Prep time: 15 minutes | Cook time: 0 minutes | Serves: 4

- 1 large cucumber, deseeded and sliced
- 4 medium tomatoes, quartered
- 1 medium red onion, thinly sliced
- ½ cup chopped fresh basil
- 3 tablespoons red wine vinegar
- 1 tablespoon extra-virgin olive oil
- ½ teaspoon Dijon mustard
- ½ teaspoon freshly ground black pepper

1. In a medium bowl, mix together the cucumber, tomatoes, red onion, and basil.
2. In a small bowl, whisk together the vinegar, olive oil, mustard, and pepper.
3. Pour the dressing over the vegetables, and gently stir until well combined.
4. Cover and chill for at least 30 minutes before serving.

Per Serving (½ cup)
calories: 72 | total carbs: 8.0g | protein: 1.0g | total fat: 4.0g | sugar: 4.0g
fiber: 1.0g | sodium: 5mg

Vegetable Deli Turkey Rolls

Prep time: 5 minutes | Cook time: 0 minutes | Serves: 4

- 4 slices nitrate-free Cajun deli turkey
- 4 teaspoons spicy mustard, divided
- 4 slices pepper Jack cheese
- ½ steak tomato, deseeded and diced
- ¼ red onion, thinly sliced
- 2 cups shredded lettuce
- ½ avocado, diced
- ¼ cup chopped banana peppers

1. On a cutting board, lay out 1 slice of deli turkey and spread with 1 teaspoon of mustard.
2. Top with 1 slice of cheese, one quarter each of the diced tomato and red onion slices, ¼ cup shredded lettuce, and one quarter each of the diced avocado and banana peppers.
3. Wrap the deli turkey tightly, but delicately, around the filling, and pin with a toothpick.
4. Repeat with the remaining ingredients, and serve.

Per Serving
calories: 152 | total carbs: 6.0g | protein: 10.0g | total fat: 9.0g | sugar: 1.0g fiber: 2.0.g | sodium: 498mg

Zucchini Fries

Prep time: 15 minutes | Cook time: 30 minutes | Serves: 6

- 3 large zucchini
- 2 large eggs
- 1 cup whole-wheat bread crumbs
- ¼ cup shredded Parmigiano-Reggiano cheese
- 1 teaspoon garlic powder
- 1 teaspoon onion powder

1. Preheat the oven to 425ºF (220ºC). Line a large rimmed baking sheet with aluminum foil.
2. Halve each zucchini lengthwise and continue slicing each piece into fries about ½ inch in diameter. You will have about 8 strips per zucchini.
3. In a small bowl, crack the eggs and beat lightly.
4. In a medium bowl, combine the bread crumbs, Parmigiano-Reggiano cheese, garlic powder, and onion powder.
5. One by one, dip each zucchini strip into the egg, then roll it in the bread crumb mixture. Put on the prepared baking sheet.
6. Roast in the preheated oven for 30 minutes, stirring the fries halfway through. Zucchini fries are done when brown and crispy.
7. Serve immediately.

Per Serving (¼ fries)
calories: 89 | total carbs: 10.0g | protein: 5.0g | total fat: 3.0g | sugar: 3.0g fiber: 1.0g | sodium: 179mg

Chapter 9
Vegetarian Dinners

87   Super Veg Chili

87   Tempeh, Mushroom and Broccoli Bowl

88   Creamy Broccoli Soup

89   Lush Roasted Vegetable Salad

90   Seitan Bites

91   Spaghetti Squash Noodles

92   Sloppy Joes in Lettuce

93   Tempeh and Avocado Lettuce Wraps

95   Zoodles with "Meat" Sauce

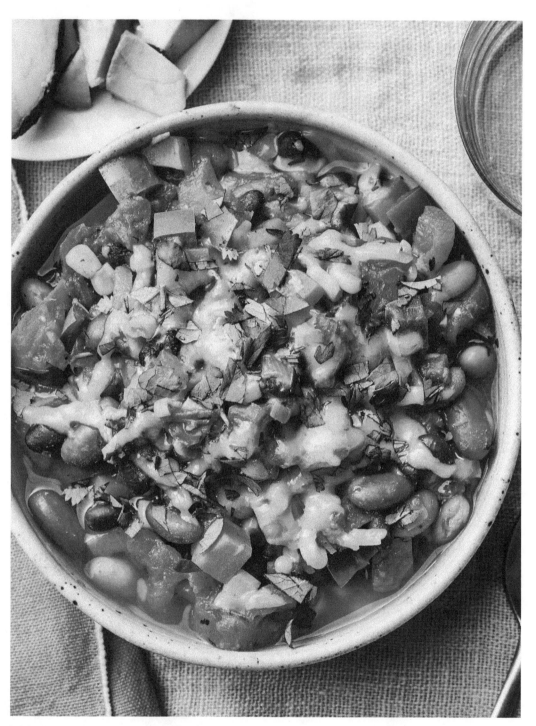

Super Veg Chili

Prep time: 10 minutes | Cook time: 40 minutes | Serves: 5

- 1 tablespoon extra-virgin olive oil
- 1 cup chopped yellow onion
- 1 cup canned diced tomatoes
- ½ cup shelled edamame
- 1 teaspoon dried cilantro
- 1 teaspoon chili powder

- 1 teaspoon ground cumin
- ¼ teaspoon salt
- 1 cup meatless soy protein crumbles
- 1 cup of water
- 8 tablespoons shredded Cheddar cheese

1. In a medium saucepan, heat the oil over medium heat. Cook the onion for 5 to 7 minutes, stirring frequently, until it is translucent.
2. Add the tomatoes and their juices, edamame, cilantro, chili powder, cumin, and salt. Cook for about 10 minutes.
3. Add the soy protein crumbles and water to the pan and cook for another 10 minutes.
4. Simmer the chili for at least 5 to 10 minutes, until chili thickens.
5. Remove from the heat and top the chili with Cheddar cheese to serve.

Per Serving (½ cup of chili plus 2 tablespoons cheese)
calories: 134 | total carbs: 9.0g | protein: 10.0g | total fat: 7.0g | sugar: 3.0g
fiber: 3.0g | sodium: 351mg

Tempeh, Mushroom and Broccoli Bowl

Prep time: 5 minutes | Cook time: 20 minutes | Serves: 5

- 8 ounces (227g) tempeh
- ½ cup water
- 4 ounces (113g) portobello mushroom, sliced in strips (1 to 2 mushrooms)
- 2 cups chopped broccoli florets

- ½ cup vegetable broth
- 1 tablespoon extra-virgin olive oil
- ¼ teaspoon dried cilantro
- ¼ teaspoon ground cumin
- ⅛ teaspoon salt

1. In a small skillet, cook the tempeh and water over medium heat for 8 to 10 minutes to soften. Remove from the skillet and set aside. Discard the water.
2. While the tempeh cooks, in a large skillet, combine the mushrooms, broccoli, and broth over medium heat. Cover and steam the vegetables for 8 to 10 minutes, until tender.
3. Once the broth has mostly evaporated, add the tempeh and oil. Mash the tempeh into small morsels and stir the vegetables and tempeh frequently while cooking for 10 minutes. Add the cilantro, cumin, and salt. Stir well and serve warm.

Per Serving (½ cup)
calories: 114 | total carbs: 8.0g | protein: 9.0g | total fat: 6.0g | sugar: 1.0g
fiber: 3.0g | sodium: 154mg

Creamy Broccoli Soup

Prep time: 10 minutes | Cook time: 20 minutes | Serves: 8

- 1 tablespoon extra-virgin olive oil
- 1 medium onion, chopped
- 1 tablespoon minced garlic
- 2 cups grated carrots
- ¼ teaspoon ground nutmeg
- ¼ cup whole-wheat pastry flour
- 2 cups low-sodium vegetable broth
- 2 cups nonfat or 1% milk
- ½ cup fat-free half-and-half
- 3 cups broccoli florets
- 2 cups shredded extra-sharp Cheddar cheese

1. In a stock pot, heat the olive oil over medium heat. Add the onion and garlic. Stir until fragrant, about 1 minute. Add the carrots and continue to stir until tender, about 2 to 3 minutes.
2. Add the nutmeg and the flour. Continue to cook, stirring constantly, until browned, 2 to 3 minutes. Add the broth and then the milk, and whisk constantly until it starts to thicken. Add the half-and-half and mix to combine well.
3. Stir in the broccoli florets. Bring to a boil and then reduce the heat to a simmer. Cook for 10 minutes or until the broccoli is tender. Use an immersion blender to purée it to a smooth consistency.
4. Stir in the Cheddar cheese until melted. Reserve some cheese as a topping for serving time.
5. Serve immediately.

Per Serving (1 cup)

calories: 193 | total carbs: 17.0g | protein: 12.0g | total fat: 9.0g | sugar: 7.0g fiber: 4.0g | sodium: 450mg

Lush Roasted Vegetable Salad

Prep time: 15 minutes | Cook time: 30 minutes | Serves: 6

- 1 small eggplant, diced
- 1 small zucchini, diced
- 1 small yellow summer squash, diced
- ½ cup grape tomatoes, halved
- 1 (15-ounce / 425-g) can chickpeas, drained and rinsed
- 3 tablespoons extra-virgin olive oil, divided
- ⅓ cup packaged quinoa
- 1 cup low-sodium vegetable or chicken broth
- 2 tablespoons freshly squeezed lemon juice
- 1 teaspoon minced fresh garlic or 1 garlic clove, minced
- 1 tablespoon dried basil
- 1 teaspoon dried oregano

1. Preheat the oven to 425°F (220°C). Line a baking sheet with parchment paper.
2. Spread the eggplant, zucchini, yellow squash, tomatoes, and chickpeas across the baking sheet and toss them with 1 tablespoon of olive oil.
3. Bake in the oven for 30 minutes, stirring once halfway through. The finished vegetables should be tender and the tomatoes should be juicy. The chickpeas will be firm and crispy.
4. While the vegetables and chickpeas are roasting, place the quinoa and broth in a small saucepan over medium-high heat. Cover and bring to a boil. Reduce the heat to low and cook for about 15 minutes, or until all liquid has absorbed. Remove the pan from the heat and fluff the quinoa with a fork.
5. In a small dish, whisk together the lemon juice, garlic, and remaining 2 tablespoons of olive oil. Mix in the basil and oregano.
6. In a large serving bowl, combine the quinoa, roasted vegetables with chickpeas, and dressing. Gently stir to combine. Serve and enjoy!

Per Serving (½ cup)
calories: 200 | total carbs: 27.0g | protein: 7.0g | total fat: 9.0g | sugar: 4.0g
fiber: 8.0g | sodium: 160mg

Seitan Bites

Prep time: 15 minutes | Cook time: 15 minutes | Makes: 8 ounces

- Nonstick cooking spray
- 1 large egg
- ½ cup flaxseed meal
- 1½ tablespoons garlic powder
- 1½ tablespoons onion powder
- 1 (8-ounce / 227-g) package seitan, cut into strips or small, 2-inch pieces
- ½ cup buffalo wing sauce

1. Preheat the oven to 350ºF (180ºC). Coat a baking sheet with cooking spray.
2. In a medium bowl, whisk the egg.
3. In another medium bowl, mix together the flaxseed meal, garlic powder, and onion powder.
4. One by one, coat each seitan piece in egg, allowing the excess egg to drip off, then lightly coat with the dry mixture.
5. Gently transfer coated pieces to the prepared baking sheet. Bake for 12 to 15 minutes, or until crispy, flipping halfway through.
6. Transfer to a large bowl, and coat with the buffalo wing sauce.
7. Serve immediately.

Per Serving
calories: 87 | total carbs: 5.0g | protein: 8.0g | total fat: 4.0g | sugar: 0g
fiber: 2.0g | sodium: 517mg

Spaghetti Squash Noodles

Prep time: 10 minutes | Cook time: 55 minutes | Serves: 3

- 1 small (3- to 4-pound / 1.4- to 1.8-kg) spaghetti squash
- ¼ cup low-sodium soy sauce
- 3 garlic cloves, minced
- 1 tablespoon oyster sauce
- 1 inch ginger root, peeled and minced
- 2 tablespoons extra-virgin olive oil
- 1 small white onion, diced
- 3 celery stalks, thinly sliced
- 2 cups shredded cabbage
- Nonstick cooking spray

1. Preheat the oven to 350ºF (180ºC). Coat a baking sheet with cooking spray.
2. Halve the spaghetti squash, remove and discard the seeds, and place the halves cut-side down on the prepared baking sheet. Bake for 30 to 45 minutes, or until the flesh is tender and can be scraped with a fork.
3. Remove from the oven, and let cool. Scrape out the flesh with a fork, creating small noodles. Set aside.
4. In a small bowl, whisk together the soy sauce, garlic, oyster sauce, and ginger.
5. In a large skillet over medium heat, heat the oil. Add the onion and celery and cook, stirring, until tender, 3 to 4 minutes. Add the cabbage and cook, stirring, until heated through, 1 to 2 minutes.
6. Add the spaghetti squash and sauce mixture. Continue cooking for another 2 minutes.
7. Serve immediately.

Per Serving

calories: 252 | total carbs: 39.0g | protein: 6.0g | total fat:11.0g
sugar: 15.0g | fiber: 9.0g | sodium: 950mg

Sloppy Joes in Lettuce

Prep time: 5 minutes | Cook time: 35 minutes | Serves: 6

- 2 cups vegetable broth
- 1 cup green lentils, well rinsed
- 1 tablespoon extra-virgin olive oil
- ½ medium yellow onion, minced
- ½ green bell pepper, minced
- 2 garlic cloves, minced
- 1 (15-ounce / 425-g) can tomato sauce
- 1 to 2 tablespoons sugar
- substitute
- 1 tablespoon Worcestershire sauce
- 2 teaspoons chili powder
- 1 teaspoon ground cumin
- 1 teaspoon paprika
- Lettuce leaves and sliced jalapeños and red onion, for serving

1. In a small saucepan over medium-high heat, combine the broth and lentils. Bring to a boil, then reduce to a simmer and cook uncovered for about 18 minutes, or until tender. Drain any excess liquid.
2. In a large skillet over medium heat, heat the oil. Add the onion, bell pepper, and garlic, and cook for 4 to 5 minutes, until tender and onions are slightly brown.
3. Add the tomato sauce, sugar substitute, Worcestershire, chili powder, cumin, paprika, and lentils. Stir to combine.
4. Continuing cooking for 5 to 10 minutes over medium heat, until warmed through and thickened.
5. Refrigerate leftovers in an airtight container. Reheat in the microwave or on the stovetop, adding extra water or broth if needed to soften.
6. Serve in lettuce leaves with sliced jalapeños and red onion.

Per Serving

calories: 163 | total carbs: 26.0g | protein: 10.0g | total fat: 3.0g | sugar: 6.0g
fiber: 11.0g | sodium: 525mg

Tempeh and Avocado Lettuce Wraps

Prep time: 10 minutes | Cook time: 30 minutes | Serves: 4

- 1 (8-ounce / 227-g) package bacon-flavored tempeh
- ¼ cup low-sodium soy sauce
- ¼ cup apple cider vinegar
- 1 teaspoon sugar substitute
- ¼ teaspoon ground cumin
- 1½ teaspoons liquid smoke
- 4 romaine lettuce leaves
- 2 teaspoons mayonnaise
- 4 tomato slices
- ½ avocado, quartered

1. Preheat the oven to 350ºF (180ºC). Line a baking sheet with parchment paper.
2. Slice the tempeh lengthwise into quarter-inch slices. You will get about 12 slices per package. It is easiest to cut the tempeh loaf in half lengthwise. Then cut each half into thirds, and then each third in half to make 12 slices.
3. To make the marinade, in a medium bowl, combine the soy sauce, vinegar, sugar substitute, cumin, and liquid smoke. Whisk well.
4. Put the tempeh in a dish, and cover with marinade. Cover and chill overnight, or at least for one hour.
5. Put the marinated tempeh strips on the prepared baking sheet.
6. Bake for 15 minutes, or until lightly brown and crispy. Flip, and bake for another 15 minutes.
7. Serve 2 strips of tempeh in each lettuce leaf with mayo, a tomato slice, and an avocado quarter.

Per Serving

calories: 129 | total carbs: 10.0g | protein: 7.0g | total fat: 7.0g | sugar: 2.0g fiber: 4.0g | sodium: 888mg

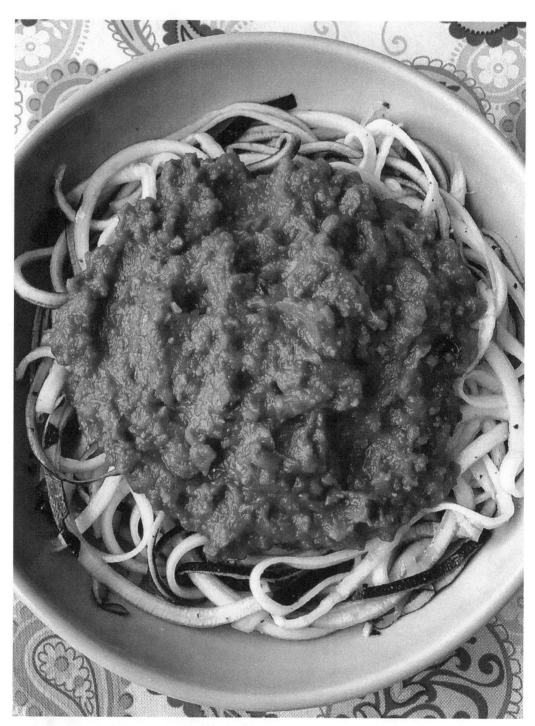

Zoodles with "Meat" Sauce

Prep time: 5 minutes | Cook time: 30 minutes | Serves: 5

For the Zoodles:
- 1 tablespoon extra-virgin olive oil
- 2 medium zucchini, peeled and spiralized

For the "Meat" Sauce:
- 1 tablespoon extra-virgin olive oil
- 1 cup soy protein crumbles
- 1 cup diced yellow onion
- 2 cups chopped tomato
- 2 teaspoons garlic powder
- 2 teaspoons Italian seasoning
- ¼ teaspoon salt
- 1 cup shredded Mozzarella cheese

To make the zoodles
1. In a large skillet, heat the oil over medium heat.
2. Put the zucchini in the skillet and cook, stirring every 30 seconds or so, for 4 to 6 minutes, until softened. Remove from the heat and place the zucchini in serving bowl.

To make the "meat" sauce
3. In the same skillet, heat the oil over medium. Add the soy protein crumbles and cook for 5 to 7 minutes. Add the onion and cook for 5 to 7 minutes, stirring frequently, or until translucent.
4. Add the tomato, garlic powder, Italian seasoning, and salt and mix well. Reduce the heat to medium-low and simmer for 7 to 10 minutes, stirring regularly, until the sauce thickens.
5. Remove from the heat and pour the sauce over zoodles. Top with Mozzarella cheese before serving.

Per Serving (¾ cup zucchini noodles plus ¾ cup sauce)
calories: 217 | total carbs: 11.0g | protein: 15.0g | total fat: 13.0g
sugar: 4.0g | fiber: 4.0g | sodium: 435mg

Chapter 10

Fish and Seafood Dinners

98   Salmon Crackers

98   Cauliflower and Shrimp Chowder

99   Creamy Parmesan and Dill Halibut

99   Lemony Sole

100   Tuna and Apple Salad

100   Scallops with Broccoli

101   Simple Salmon Roast

101   Shrimp and Vegetable Salad

103   Cod en Papillote

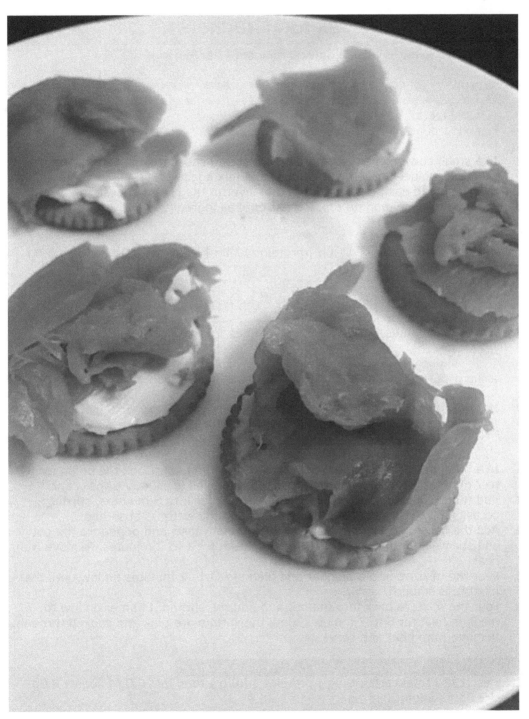

Salmon Crackers

Prep time: 15 minutes | Cook time: 0 minutes | Serves: 4

- ½ cup very thinly sliced red onion
- ⅓ cup whipped cream cheese
- ¼ cup capers
- Freshly ground black pepper
- 24 whole-wheat crackers
- 12 ounces (340 g) smoked salmon, sliced

1. In a small bowl, combine the red onion, cream cheese, and capers, then stir well to combine. Season with pepper and mix again.
2. Evenly spread each cracker with a thin layer of the cream cheese mixture.
3. Lay a piece of salmon on top. Repeat until all ingredients are used. Serve.

Per Serving
calories: 192 | total carbs: 11.0g | protein: 17.0g | total fat: 8.0g | sugar: 2.0g
fiber: 2.0g | sodium: 2091mg

Cauliflower and Shrimp Chowder

Prep time: 10 minutes | Cook time: 25 minutes | Serves: 4

- 1 tablespoon extra-virgin olive oil
- 1 cup diced yellow onion
- 1 cup cauliflower rice
- ½ cup water
- ¼ teaspoon salt
- ½ cup unsweetened light canned
- coconut milk
- ½ unsweetened almond milk
- 4 tablespoons nutritional yeast
- Dash freshly ground black pepper
- 1½ cups peeled raw small salad shrimp

1. In a medium saucepan, heat the oil over medium heat. Cook the onion for 5 to 7 minutes, stirring frequently, or until the onion is slightly translucent.
2. Add the cauliflower rice, water, and salt. Cook for 6 to 8 minutes, stirring occasionally, until cauliflower is softened and the water is absorbed.
3. Add the coconut milk, almond milk, nutritional yeast, and pepper to the pot and stir well. Simmer on low-to-medium heat for 1 to 2 minutes. Remove from heat.
4. Pour the mixture into a blender and blend for 1 to 2 minutes on low until the mixture is smooth.
5. Pour the mixture back into the pot and add the shrimp. Simmer on low to medium heat for 5 to 7 minutes, until the shrimp are pink and cooked through. Remove from heat and serve.

Per Serving (6 tablespoons shrimp plus ½ cup chowder)
calories: 133 | total carbs: 6.0g | protein: 14.0.g | total fat: 6.0g | sugar: 3.0g
fiber: 3.0g | sodium: 358mg

Creamy Parmesan and Dill Halibut

Prep time: 5 minutes | Cook time: 20 minutes | Serves: 4

- 4 (6-ounce / 170-g) fresh halibut fillets (1-inch thick)
- Juice of ½ lemon
- Salt, to taste
- Freshly ground black pepper, to taste
- 1/3 cup low-fat sour cream
- 1/3 cup low-fat, plain Greek yogurt
- 1/3 cup Parmesan cheese
- ½ teaspoon garlic powder
- ½ teaspoon dried dill
- 3 scallions, finely chopped

1. Preheat the oven to 400°F (205ºC).
2. Put the halibut fillets in a large baking dish, and add the lemon juice. Season with salt and pepper.
3. In a small bowl, mix the sour cream, yogurt, cheese, garlic powder, dill, and scallions. Spread the mixture over the fish.
4. Bake in the oven for 15 to 20 minutes, or until the internal temperature reaches 145ºF (63ºC), the fish is opaque and flakes easily with a fork, and the cheese is golden, and serve.

Per Serving

calories: 345 | total carbs: 6.0g | protein: 52.0.g | total fat: 12.0g | sugar: 2.0g fiber: 2.0g | sodium: 293mg

Lemony Sole

Prep time: 5 minutes | Cook time: 20 minutes | Serves: 4

- ¼ cup whole-wheat flour
- Salt, to taste
- Freshly ground black pepper, to taste
- 1 pound (454 g) boneless, skinless
- sole fillets
- 1 tablespoon extra-virgin olive oil
- 1 tablespoon melted butter
- Juice of 2 lemons, divided

1. On a large plate, pour the flour and season with salt and pepper. Lightly dredge the sole fillets in the flour mixture and set aside.
2. In a small bowl, combine the olive oil, melted butter, and half the lemon juice. Mix well.
3. Heat a large nonstick pan over medium-high heat and add half the oil-butter mixture. Allow it to warm through for about 1 minute.
4. Put half the fish in the pan and cook for about 5 minutes, then flip and cook another 2 minutes, or until the fish is cooked through and flakes very easily. Repeat with the remaining oil-butter mixture and fish.
5. Plate the fish and top with the remaining lemon juice. Serve.

Per Serving

calories: 180 | total carbs: 8.0g | protein: 21.0g | total fat: 8.0g | sugar: 1.0g fiber: 1.0g | sodium: 103mg

Tuna and Apple Salad

Prep time: 10 minutes | Cook time: 0 minutes | Serves: 4

- 3 (5-ounce / 142-g) cans water-packed albacore tuna, drained
- ¼ cup low-fat mayonnaise
- 1 medium Granny Smith apple, peeled and finely chopped
- ¼ cup finely diced red onion
- Salt, to taste
- Freshly ground black pepper, to taste

1. In a large bowl, combine the tuna and mayonnaise. Using a fork, mix well.
2. Add the apple and red onion and toss again to combine.
3. Season with salt and pepper. Serve at room temperature or chilled.

Per Serving
calories: 118 | total carbs: 11.0g | protein: 17.0g | total fat: 3.0g | sugar: 5.0g fiber: 3.0g | sodium: 401mg

Scallops with Broccoli

Prep time: 5 minutes | Cook time: 10 minutes | Serves: 4

- 1 pound (454 g) raw jumbo sea scallops
- 1 tablespoon garlic powder
- ½ teaspoon freshly ground black pepper
- ⅛ teaspoon salt
- 2 tablespoons extra-virgin olive oil
- 2 cups chopped broccoli florets
- ¼ cup water

1. Blot the scallops dry with a paper towel.
2. In a small bowl, mix the garlic powder, pepper, and salt and set aside.
3. Coat a large skillet with the oil and heat over medium-high heat.
4. One at a time, lightly dab each scallop with the spice mixture on both flat sides. Put the scallop in the skillet. Repeat with remaining scallops.
5. Cook the scallops for 2 minutes on each side. Remove the scallops to a plate and set aside.
6. Lower the heat to medium and place the broccoli in the skillet. Add the water, cover, and steam for 3 to 5 minutes, or until the broccoli is tender. Drain the broccoli and sprinkle with salt and pepper to taste.
7. Serve the scallops over the broccoli.

Per Serving (3 or 4 scallops plus ½ cup broccoli)
calories: 164 | total carbs: 8.0g | protein: 9.0.g | total fat: 8.0g | sugar: 1.0g fiber: 1.0g | sodium: 236mg

Simple Salmon Roast

Prep time: 15 minutes | Cook time: 20 minutes | Serves: 2

- 2 (4-ounce / 113-g) salmon fillets
- 2 tablespoons honey-mustard
- 2 garlic cloves, crushed
- Juice of ½ lemon
- ½ teaspoon smoked paprika
- 1 tablespoon snipped fresh chives
- Salt and freshly ground black pepper, to taste
- Cooking spray

1. Preheat the oven to 400°F (205°C).
2. Spray a rimmed baking sheet with cooking spray. Put the salmon on the baking sheet. Mix the mustard with the garlic, lemon juice, paprika, chives, and salt and pepper. Brush over the salmon.
3. Roast for 15 to 20 minutes, until cooked through and browned. Serve hot.

Per Serving

calories: 192 | total carbs: 3.1g | protein: 24.3g | total fat: 8.8g | sugar: 0.6g fiber: 1.0g | sodium: 664mg

Shrimp and Vegetable Salad

Prep time: 5 minutes | Cook time: 20 minutes | Serves: 4

- Nonstick cooking spray
- ¼ cup diced yellow or red onion
- ¼ cup diced bell pepper
- 2 teaspoons extra-virgin olive oil, divided
- 1½ cups canned baby shrimp
- 2 tablespoons nonfat plain Greek yogurt
- 1 teaspoon apple cider vinegar
- ½ teaspoon garlic powder
- ½ teaspoon ground cumin

1. Preheat the oven to 400°F (205ºC). Line a baking sheet with parchment paper or aluminum foil and spritz with nonstick cooking spray.
2. Arrange the onion and pepper on the baking sheet and drizzle with 1 tablespoon of oil. Toss the vegetables with the oil and coat well. Bake for about 20 minutes, until all the vegetables are softened and lightly browned. Remove from heat.
3. In a large mixing bowl, combine the onion and pepper with the shrimp, yogurt, remaining oil, vinegar, garlic powder, and cumin.
4. Serve warm or chill in the refrigerator before serving.

Per Serving (½ CUP)

calories: 71 | total carbs: 2.0g | protein: 10.0.g | total fat: 3.0g | sugar: 1.0g fiber: 1.0g | sodium: 189mg

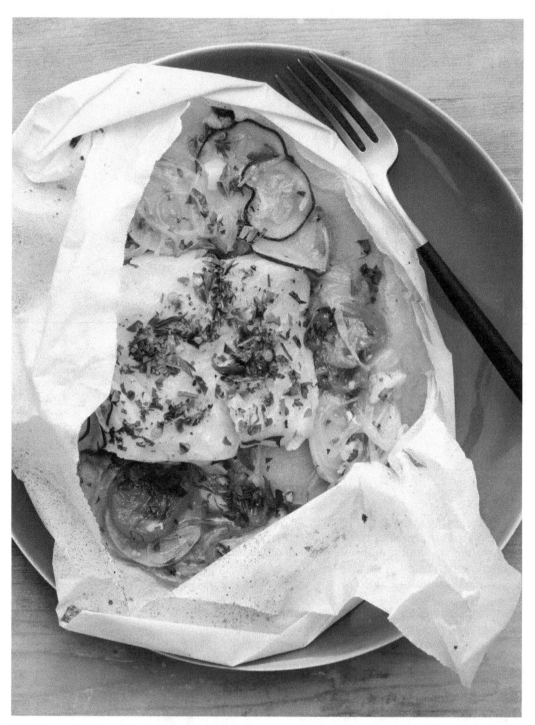

Cod en Papillote

Prep time: 15 minutes | Cook time: 15 minutes | Serves: 4

- 2 teaspoons extra-virgin olive oil
- 2 garlic cloves, minced
- 1 shallot, thinly sliced
- ¼ cup dry white wine
- 1 tablespoon freshly squeezed lemon juice
- 4 (6-ounce / 170-g) boneless cod fillets
- Salt, to taste
- Freshly ground black pepper, to taste
- 1 pint cherry tomatoes
- ½ cup chopped fresh basil

1. Preheat the oven to 400°F (205ºC).
2. In a small saucepan over medium heat, heat the oil. Add the garlic and shallot, and sauté until the shallot is softened and the garlic is fragrant, 3 to 5 minutes. Add the white wine and lemon juice, and bring to a gentle simmer. Remove from the heat, and let cool.
3. Season the cod fillets with salt and pepper.
4. Lay out a sheet of parchment paper with a long side facing you. Put one cod fillet in the middle of the paper, and pile with a quarter of the tomatoes and a quarter of the basil.
5. Bring the two long ends of the paper together and begin folding in small increments until tightly sealed. Then, roll and tightly crimp the open ends.
6. Open the paper back up, as the fold lines have now been established, and pour in ¼ of the lemon-garlic liquid. Refold the paper so that no steam can escape. Repeat with the 3 remaining fillets.
7. Transfer the packets to a baking sheet, and bake for 10 to 15 minutes, or until the fish is opaque and flakes easily with a fork.
8. Remove from the oven and allow to rest for 5 minutes before serving.
9. Serve warm.

Per Serving

calories: 194 | total carbs: 5.0g | protein: 31.0g | total fat: 3.0g | sugar: 2.0g
fiber: 1.0g | sodium: 126mg

Chapter 11

Poultry Dinners

106   Artichoke and Spinach Chicken Rolls

107   Salsa Verde Chicken Bowl

108   Veg and Chicken Meatballs

109   Avocado Turkey Blt

109   Turkey and Spinach Burgers

110   BBQ Chicken with Avocado

110   Chicken and Water Chestnut Wraps

111   Cucumber Turkey Rolls

111   Mexican Salsa Chicken

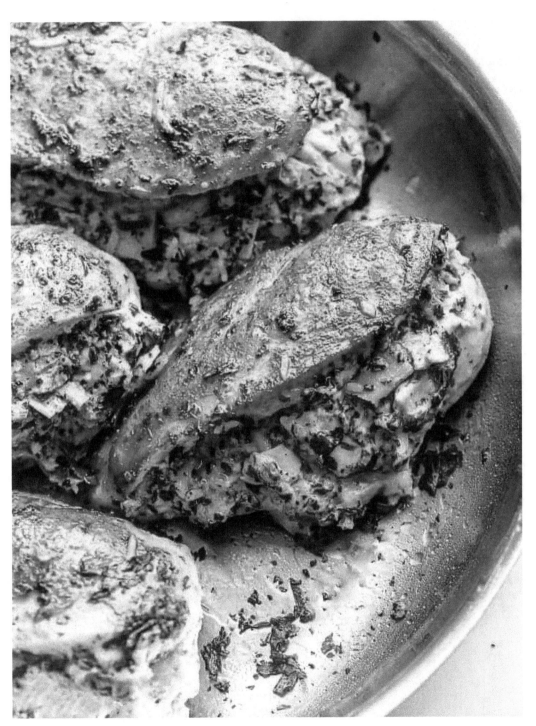

Artichoke and Spinach Chicken Rolls

Prep time: 10 minutes | Cook time: 25 minutes | Serves 4

- ½ teaspoon extra-virgin olive oil
- 4 cups baby spinach
- 4 (4-ounce / 113-g) boneless, skinless chicken breasts
- ½ cup ricotta cheese
- 1 (6-ounce / 170-g) jar marinated

- artichoke hearts, drained
- Salt and freshly ground black pepper, to taste
- ¼ cup white wine
- Nonstick cooking spray

1. Preheat the oven to 375ºF (190ºC). Spray an oven-safe casserole dish with cooking spray.
2. In a medium skillet over low heat, warm the olive oil. Sauté the baby spinach.
3. While the spinach cooks, pound the chicken breasts with a rolling pin until you're left with thin cutlets.
4. In a blender or food processor, pulse the ricotta cheese and artichoke hearts, then transfer the mixture to a bowl.
5. Remove the cooked spinach from the skillet and add it to the cheese mixture. Stir to combine.
6. Put the chicken on a flat surface, then spoon the cheese mixture on top of each cutlet. Roll the chicken to enclose the filling and place seam-side down in the casserole dish. Repeat until all the chicken is rolled.
7. Lightly coat the top of each chicken roll with cooking spray and season with salt and pepper.
8. Pour the white wine into the casserole dish so that it coats the bottom, then cover the dish with aluminum foil. Bake for about 25 minutes, or until the chicken is fully cooked and juices run clear. Serve hot.

Per Serving
calories: 215 | total carbs: 6.0g | protein: 28.0g | total fat: 8.0g | sugar: 1.0g fiber: 1.0g | sodium: 389mg

Salsa Verde Chicken Bowl

Prep time: 5 minutes | Cook time: 20 minutes | Serves 4

- 3 (6-ounce / 170-g) boneless, skinless chicken breasts, each cut into 4 pieces
- 4 cups water, plus 2 tablespoons
- 1 (1-pound / 454-g) package frozen cauliflower rice
- 1 tablespoon extra-virgin olive oil
- 1 (12-ounce / 340-g) jar tomatillo salsa
- 1 avocado, peeled, pitted, and diced
- 1 limes, quartered, for serving

1. In a heavy-bottomed pan over high heat, add the chicken with 4 cups water and bring to a boil. When the water is just boiling, reduce the heat to medium-low, cover with a lid, and cook for about 10 minutes, or until the chicken is fully cooked and no longer pink.
2. While the chicken cooks, in a nonstick pan over medium heat, add the cauliflower rice, olive oil, and the remaining 2 tablespoons of water. Stir to combine and cook for about 5 minutes, until the rice is just softened or the water has evaporated.
3. Once the chicken is cooked, drain the water and let the chicken cool slightly.
4. Put the chicken in a blender or food processor and pulse to shred it into small pieces. Alternatively, you can shred the chicken by hand with two forks.
5. In the same pan used to cook the chicken, over medium heat, add the shredded chicken and salsa and mix to combine. Cook for about 5 minutes, or until the mixture is hot.
6. Plate the dish with the cauliflower rice first, topped with the shredded chicken, avocado, and 1 or 2 quarters of lime.

`Per Serving`
calories: 292 | total carbs: 15.0g | protein: 29.0g | total fat: 13.0g | sugar: 6.0g
fiber: 9.0g | sodium: 724mg

Veg and Chicken Meatballs

Prep time: 5 minutes | Cook time: 25 minutes | Serves 4

- 1 medium zucchini, shredded
- 1 large carrot, shredded
- ¼ cup honey mustard
- 4 garlic cloves, minced
- Salt and freshly ground black
- pepper, to taste
- 1 pound (454 g) lean ground chicken
- Nonstick cooking spray

1. Preheat the oven to 375ºF (190ºC). Spray a baking sheet with cooking spray and set aside.
2. In a colander, drain the shredded zucchini and carrot and press out any residual liquid.
3. In a large bowl, combine the drained zucchini and carrot mixture with the honey mustard and garlic. Season with salt and pepper and stir to combine.
4. Add the chicken to the vegetable mixture and mix to combine, being careful not to overmix. Using an ice cream scoop, portion out 2-inch meatballs onto the prepared baking sheet.
5. Bake for 20 to 25 minutes, flipping 15 minutes into cooking, until the meatballs are fully cooked and their internal temperature has reached 165ºF (74ºC).
6. Serve immediately.

Per Serving
calories: 254 | total carbs: 22.0g | protein: 23.0g | total fat: 9.0g | sugar: 19.0g
fiber: 1.0g | sodium: 154mg

Avocado Turkey Blt

Prep time: 15 minutes | Cook time: 15 minutes | Serves 4

- 8 slices turkey bacon
- 1 head iceberg lettuce
- 1 medium avocado, peeled, pitted, and mashed
- Freshly ground black pepper, to taste
- 1 pound (454 g) deli-sliced turkey
- 1 large tomato, thinly sliced

1. Preheat the oven to 400ºF (205ºC).
2. Put the turkey bacon on a baking sheet and cook for about 10 minutes, then flip and cook about 5 more minutes, or until crispy. Remove and set aside to cool.
3. While the turkey bacon cooks, slicing the root end off the head of lettuce and separating the leaves.
4. To assemble each wrap, stack 2 lettuce leaves on top of one another, spread a thin layer of avocado on top, then season with freshly ground pepper.
5. Layer 2 or 3 slices of turkey, 2 slices of tomato, and 1 slice of crispy turkey bacon, then roll the lettuce wraps and serve immediately.

Per Serving

calories: 291 | total carbs: 18.0g | protein: 28.0g | total fat: 13.0g | sugar: 10.0g
fiber: 5.0g | sodium: 1342mg

Turkey and Spinach Burgers

Prep time: 5 minutes | Cook time: 25 minutes | Serves 4

- 1 small white onion, diced
- $\frac{1}{3}$ cup crumbled feta
- 2 tablespoons chopped fresh dill
- 3 teaspoons extra-virgin olive oil, divided
- Salt and freshly ground black pepper, to taste
- 3 cups baby spinach
- 1 pound (454 g) lean ground turkey
- Nonstick cooking spray

1. Preheat the oven to 375ºF (190ºC). Spray a baking sheet with cooking spray and set aside.
2. In a large bowl, mix the onion, feta, dill, and 1 teaspoon olive oil. Season the mixture with salt and pepper and stir to combine.
3. In a medium skillet over low heat, warm the remaining 2 teaspoons olive oil. Sauté the spinach for about 5 minutes, or until just wilted. Set aside to cool.
4. Chop the spinach roughly and add to the onion mixture. Stir to combine.
5. Add the ground turkey and mix until just combined. Do not overmix. Using clean hands, form the mixture into 4 burgers.
6. Put the burgers on the prepared baking sheet and bake for about 10 minutes, then flip and bake another 10 minutes, until fully cooked and the internal temperature reaches 165ºF (74ºC). Serve hot.

Per Serving

calories: 197 | total carbs: 3.0g | protein: 29.0g | total fat: 8.0g | sugar: 2.0g
fiber: 1.0g | sodium: 235mg

BBQ Chicken with Avocado

Prep time: 5 minutes | Cook time: 25 minutes | Serves 4

- ½ cup low-sugar barbecue sauce
- 2 tablespoons water
- Nonstick cooking spray
- 1 pound (454 g) boneless, skinless chicken breasts
- 1 medium avocado, peeled and pitted
- ¼ cup apple cider vinegar
- 1 (14-ounce / 397-g) bag coleslaw mix

1. Preheat the oven to 375ºF (190ºC).
2. In a small bowl, combine the barbecue sauce and water.
3. Spray a small baking dish with cooking spray, then add the chicken.
4. Using a brush to coat the chicken with the barbecue sauce.
5. Cover the dish with aluminum foil and bake for 20 to 25 minutes, until cooked through.
6. While the chicken is cooking, mash together the avocado and vinegar, then add the mixture to the coleslaw mix. Toss well to combine and set aside.
7. When the chicken has an internal temperature of 165ºF (74ºC), remove from the oven. Serve the chicken on a bed of coleslaw.

Per Serving

calories: 221 | total carbs: 13.0g | protein: 25.0g | total fat: 9.0g | sugar: 6.0g
fiber: 5.0g | sodium: 591mg

Chicken and Water Chestnut Wraps

Prep time: 10 minutes | Cook time: 15 minutes | Serves 4

- 1 tablespoon sesame oil
- 1 pound (454 g) lean ground chicken
- 1 head butter lettuce
- 1 (8-ounce / 227-g) can water
- chestnuts, drained and roughly chopped
- ¼ cup hoisin sauce

1. In a large skillet over medium heat, warm the sesame oil, then add the chicken.
2. While the chicken is cooking, prepare the lettuce by removing the leaves from the head and setting them aside.
3. Add the water chestnuts to the chicken and stir to combine. Add the hoisin sauce and break up the chicken into smaller pieces.
4. Cook for about 15 minutes, or until the internal temperature of the chicken reaches at least 165ºF (74ºC).
5. When the chicken is finished cooking, fill each lettuce wrap with the chicken mixture, fold like tacos, and serve.

Per Serving

calories: 263 | total carbs: 14.0g | protein: 23.0g | total fat: 13.0g | sugar: 12.0g
fiber: 2.0g | sodium: 399mg

Cucumber Turkey Rolls

Prep time: 10 minutes | Cook time: 0 minutes | Serves 4

- 8 Kirby cucumbers
- 1 large carrot, peeled
- 1 pound (454 g) deli-sliced turkey
- 8 ounces (227 g) thinly sliced

- Cheddar cheese
- ½ cup grainy mustard
- Freshly ground black pepper, to taste

1. Halve each cucumber lengthwise and set aside.
2. Using a vegetable peeler, peel the carrot into thin and pliable ribbons and set aside.
3. On 2 slices of turkey, place ½ slice of cheese, topped with mustard, a sprinkle of pepper, and a few carrot strips.
4. Put 1 cucumber half on top and roll the turkey around the cucumber. Plate the roll seam-side down or use a toothpick to secure the seam.
5. Repeat until all cucumbers are used. Serve cold.

Per Serving
calories: 392 | total carbs: 14.0g | protein: 35.0g | total fat: 23.0g | sugar: 8.0g
fiber: 2.0g | sodium: 1421mg

Mexican Salsa Chicken

Prep time: 5 minutes | Cook time: 45 minutes | Serves 4

- 1 (12-ounce / 340-g) jar salsa
- 1 pound (454 g) boneless, skinless chicken breast, pounded until about ½-inch thick
- 1 (12-ounce / 340-g) can fat-free refried beans

- 1 medium white onion, sliced
- Salt and freshly ground black pepper, to taste
- ¾ cup shredded Cheddar cheese
- Nonstick cooking spray

1. Preheat the oven to 350ºF (180ºC).
2. Coat a casserole dish with cooking spray and spread half of the salsa on the bottom of the pan. Put the chicken on the salsa and spread the refried beans atop the chicken. Add a layer of onion, followed by the remaining salsa, then season with salt and pepper.
3. Evenly sprinkle the cheese over the top and cover with aluminum foil. Bake for 35 minutes, or until the chicken is cooked through and juices run clear.
4. Remove the foil and bake for another 10 minutes, until the cheese is just golden brown. Serve hot.

Per Serving
calories: 313 | total carbs: 24.0g | protein: 34.0g | total fat: 10.0g | sugar: 5.0g
fiber: 8.0g | sodium: 1135mg

Chapter 12

Pork and Beef Dinners

114   Pork Tenderloin Asian Style

114   Creamy Horseradish London Broil

115   Apple Braised Pork

115   Beef and mushroom Stroganoff

116   Madeira Pork Tenderloin

116   Pork Medallions with Mushrooms

117   Beef Brisket Roast

118   Ritzy Beef and Veg Stir-fry

119   Hearty Beef Bordelaise

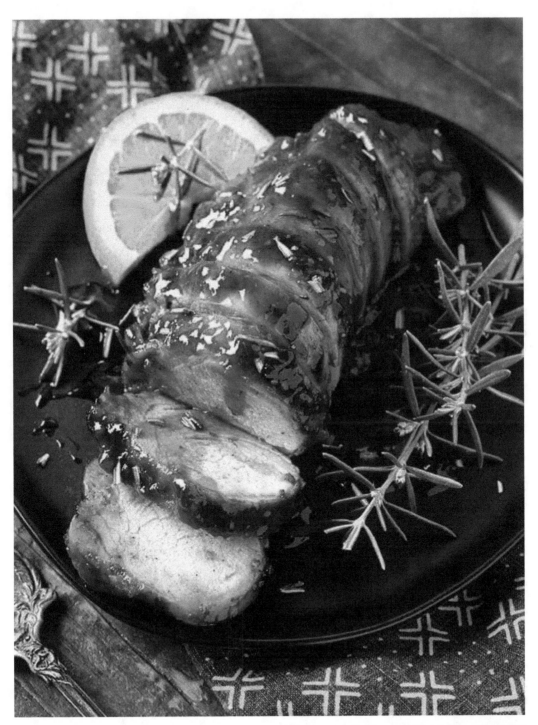

Pork Tenderloin Asian Style

Prep time: 10 minutes | Cook time: 35 minutes | Serves 4

- 2 pounds (907 g) pork tenderloin
- 2 tablespoons Worcestershire sauce
- 1/3 cup soy sauce (light)
- 4 cloves garlic, minced
- 2 tablespoons rice vinegar
- 2 tablespoons lemon juice
- 1 tablespoon ginger
- 1/3 cup brown sugar
- 1 tablespoon dry mustard
- 1½ teaspoons ground black pepper

1. Combine all the ingredients in a resealable plastic bag. Toss to coat the pork tenderloin well. Refrigerate overnight.
2. Preheat the oven to 375ºF (190ºC).
3. Remove the pork from the marinade and transfer to a baking pan. Pour the marinade over.
4. Arrange the pan in the oven and bake for 35 minutes or until the pork is well browned. Flip the pork halfway through.
5. Serve warm.

Per Serving
calories: 399 | total carbs: 27.7g | protein: 49.6g | total fat: 9.0g | sugar: 23.1g
fiber: 1.0g | sodium: 574mg

Creamy Horseradish London Broil

Prep time: 6 minutes | Cook time: 10 minutes | Serves 4

- 1 pound (454 g) lean London broil (top round or flank steak)
- 1½ teaspoons garlic powder
- 1 tablespoon lemon pepper
- ½ cup fat-free sour cream
- 1 tablespoon concentrated beef broth
- 2 tablespoons prepared horseradish

1. Preheat broiler and arrange rack to top position.
2. With a sharp knife, score top of London broil to keep it from curling. Sprinkle with garlic powder and lemon-pepper.
3. Put in a nonstick broiling pan and broil for 4 minutes on each side for medium rare.
4. While steak is broiling, combine sour cream, concentrated beef broth, and horseradish in a small bowl.
5. Slice the steak thinly on diagonal, pour the sauce over it, and serve.

Per Serving
calories: 182 | total carbs: 8.0g | protein: 28.0g | total fat: 5.0g | sugar: 8.0g
fiber: 0g | sodium: 723mg

Apple Braised Pork

Prep time: 10 minutes | Cook time: 30 minutes | Serves 4

- 1 pound (454 g) pork tenderloin
- 2 garlic cloves, minced
- ¼ teaspoon ground nutmeg
- 1 tablespoon ground fresh grated ginger
- 1 large onion, cut into ½-inch wedges
- 2 medium Granny Smith apples, peeled, cored, and cut into ½-inch wedges
- 2 packets Splenda
- ½ teaspoon ground cinnamon
- ½ cup water
- Cooking spray

1. Preheat the oven to 350ºF (180ºC). Spritz a baking pan with cooking spray. Put pork tenderloin in the baking pan.
2. In a small bowl, combine garlic, nutmeg, and ginger and rub onto pork.
3. Surround tenderloin with alternating wedges of onion and apple. Spray onion and apple wedges with cooking spray, sprinkle with sweetener and cinnamon, and pour water over onions and apples.
4. Cover with foil and bake for 20 minutes. Remove foil and bake for 10 minutes more.
5. Slice meat thinly and serve.

Per Serving
calories: 233 | total carbs: 17.0g | protein: 24.0g | total fat: 7.0g | sugar: 14.0g
fiber: 3.0g | sodium: 56mg

Beef and mushroom Stroganoff

Prep time: 10 minutes | Cook time: 1 hour 30 minutes | Serves 4

- 2 garlic cloves, minced
- 1 pound (454 g) lean eye round, cut into 1-inch cubes
- 1 (6-ounce / 170-g) can tomato sauce
- ½ cup dry red wine
- 1 cup sliced fresh mushrooms
- 1 bay leaf
- ½ cup fat-free sour cream
- Salt and ground black pepper, to taste
- Butter-flavored cooking spray

1. Coat bottom of large nonstick lidded skillet with cooking spray and heat over medium-high heat until hot. Sauté garlic for 1 minute until soft. Add meat and brown, stirring, for 3 minutes.
2. Add tomato sauce, wine, mushrooms, and bay leaf and lower heat. Simmer, covered, over low heat for 1½ hours.
3. Turn off heat and stir in sour cream. Add salt and pepper. Serve immediately.

Per Serving
calories: 229 | total carbs: 10.0g | protein: 27.0g | total fat: 4.0g | sugar: 9.0g
fiber: 1.0g | sodium: 254mg

Madeira Pork Tenderloin

Prep time: 10 minutes | Cook time: 18 minutes | Serves 4

- 1 tablespoon olive oil
- 1 pound (454 g) pork tenderloin
- ¾ cup thinly sliced shallots
- ¾ cup Madeira wine
- ¼ teaspoon vanilla extract
- 2 tablespoons balsamic vinegar
- Brown-sugar artificial sweetener (1 teaspoon equivalent)
- Salt and ground black pepper, to taste

1. Slice the tenderloin into ½-inch slices.
2. In a large nonstick skillet, heat the olive oil and sauté the pork over medium heat for 4 minutes, turning once. Remove from pan and keep warm.
3. Add shallots to pan and sauté for 3 minutes.
4. Add wine and vanilla to pan, stirring to scrape up any browned bits. Lower heat and simmer for 10 minutes, or until liquid is reduced slightly.
5. Stir in balsamic vinegar and sweetener, return pork and any accumulated juices to pan, and turn once to coat. Add salt and pepper to taste.

Per Serving

calories: 259 | total carbs: 12.0g | protein: 24.0g | total fat: 7.0g | sugar: 14.0g
fiber: 0g | sodium: 176mg

Pork Medallions with Mushrooms

Prep time: 10 minutes | Cook time: 8 minutes | Serves 4

- 1 pound (454 g) pork tenderloin, sliced into ½-inch slices
- 1 tablespoon olive oil
- ½ cup thinly sliced shallots
- 1 cup thinly sliced fresh mushrooms
- ½ cup dry white wine
- 2 tablespoons concentrated chicken broth
- ¼ teaspoon dried thyme
- 2 teaspoons whole-grain mustard
- ¼ cup fat-free sour cream
- Salt and ground black pepper, to taste

1. In a medium nonstick skillet, heat the olive oil over medium-high heat until hot but not smoking. Brown pork on both sides, then lower heat and sauté for 3 minutes, until cooked through. Remove the pork from pan.
2. Re-spray the pan and sauté shallots and mushrooms, stirring until lightly browned.
3. Stir in wine, scraping up any browned bits. Add concentrated chicken broth and thyme and simmer for 2 minutes.
4. Stir in mustard and sour cream and simmer for 1 to 2 minutes. Add pork and any accumulated meat juices and turn pork to coat. Add salt and pepper to taste.

Per Serving

calories: 232 | total carbs: 8.0g | protein: 25.0g | total fat: 8.0g | sugar: 8.0g
fiber: 0g | sodium: 521mg

Beef Brisket Roast

Prep time: 15 minutes | Cook time: 2 hours 10 minutes | Serves 8

- 2 tablespoons olive oil
- 2 pounds (907 g) lean beef brisket
- 1½ cups coarsely chopped onion
- 2 garlic cloves, minced
- 2 tablespoons sweet paprika
- 1 (14.5-ounce / 411-g) can low-sodium beef broth
- 1 cup strong brewed coffee
- 1 cup water
- 2 tablespoons concentrated beef broth
- 2 bay leaves
- 1 ounce (28 g) dried mushrooms
- 1½ cups coarsely chopped carrot
- ¾ pound (340 g) green beans, ends trimmed
- Salt and ground black pepper, to taste

1. In a nonstick Dutch oven, heat the olive oil over medium-high heat until hot but not smoking. Put meat in Dutch oven and brown on both sides, about 5 minutes. Remove meat from pot and pour off accumulated fat.
2. Put onion, garlic, and paprika in pot, stir, cover, and cook over medium heat for 5 to 7 minutes, or until onion is softened.
3. Add meat back to pot on top of onion mixture and pour in beef broth, coffee, and water. Stir in concentrated beef broth, and bring to a boil. Then, add bay leaves, mushrooms, and carrot, lower heat to a simmer, cover, and cook for 1½ hours.
4. Remove meat from pot and slice thinly on diagonal.
5. Add meat back to pot, place green beans on top, cover, and cook for another 30 minutes. Add salt and pepper to taste.

Per Serving

calories: 231 | total carbs: 11.0g | protein: 27.0g | total fat: 9.0g | sugar: 8.0g
fiber: 3.0g | sodium: 681mg

Ritzy Beef and Veg Stir-fry

Prep time: 20 minutes | Cook time: 15 minutes | Serves 4

- ⅓ cup low-sodium soy sauce
- 2 tablespoons rice vinegar
- ¼ cup dry sherry
- 1 teaspoon minced fresh ginger
- 1 teaspoon sesame oil
- 2 packets Splenda
- Cooking spray
- 1 pound (454 g) lean beef, sliced thinly
- 1 large sweet onion, peeled, cut in half, and sliced into ¼-inch slices
- 1 clove garlic, minced
- 2 scallions or green onions (white and green parts), sliced into ¼-inch slices
- 1 red, yellow, or orange bell pepper, deseeded and cut into ¼-inch slices
- 4 large white mushrooms, sliced
- 1 medium zucchini, cut into ¼ inch rounds
- ½ pound (227 g) snow peas, stringed, cut in half diagonally
- ½ head bok choy, rinsed, sliced on the diagonal into ½-inch slices

1. To make sauce: In a saucepan, combine all sauce ingredients and bring to a simmer.
2. Spray cooking spray in a skillet, then heat over medium-high heat until it shimmers. Add sliced beef and stir-fry for 2 minutes, or until barely browned. Remove beef from pan and keep warm.
3. Wipe pan, re-spray, and heat until shimmering. Add onion and garlic and cook, stirring, for about 4 minutes, or until translucent, but do not brown.
4. Stir in scallions, peppers, mushrooms, and zucchini. Add sauce and cook, stirring, for 3 to 4 minutes.
5. Stir in peas and bok choy, cover, and steam for 2 minutes.
6. Stir beef back into pan and cook for 2 minutes, or until heated through.

Per Serving

calories: 334 | total carbs: 23.0g | protein: 27.0g | total fat: 12.0g | sugar: 19.0g
fiber: 4.0g | sodium: 899mg

Hearty Beef Bordelaise

Prep time: 15 minutes | Cook time: 2 hours 15 minutes | Serves 4

- 1 tablespoon olive oil
- 1 pound (454 g) lean beef round, trimmed and cut into 1-inch cubes
- 1½ cups chopped onion
- 2 large garlic cloves, chopped
- ½ cup dry red wine
- ½ cup fat-free, low-sodium beef broth
- 1 cup chopped tomato
- 1 (6-ounce / 170-g) can tomato juice
- 1 piece orange peel
- 1 teaspoon Worcestershire sauce
- 1 teaspoon chopped fresh rosemary, or ½ teaspoon dried
- ½ pound (227 g) peeled baby carrots

1. In a heavy pot, heat the olive oil over medium-high heat until hot but not smoking. Brown beef on all sides and transfer to a bowl.
2. Discard any fat accumulated in pot. Add onion and garlic to pot and cook over medium heat, stirring, for 2 minutes, or until golden.
3. Add wine, broth, tomato, tomato juice, orange peel, Worcestershire, and rosemary to pot and bring to a boil. Add back to pot beef and any meat juices that have accumulated.
4. Cover and lower heat; simmer for 30 minutes.
5. Stir in carrots, cover, and simmer for 1½ hours.
6. Uncover, increase heat to medium-high, and cook for 15 minutes, or until liquid in pot reduces and is slightly thickened.

Per Serving

calories: 244 | total carbs: 16.0g | protein: 27.0g | total fat: 4.0g | sugar: 13.0g
fiber: 3.0g | sodium: 133mg

Chapter 13

Sweets and Treats

122   Lemon Curd Mini Cake

122   Cheesy Berry Compote

123   Berry, Mango, and Kiwi Cake

123   Super Easy Chocolate Mousse

124   Fig and Orange Cheesecake

124   Gelatin Cottage Cheese

125   Peanut Butter Oat Cookies

125   Rhubarb Apple Popsicles

127   Toffee Apple Protein Crumble

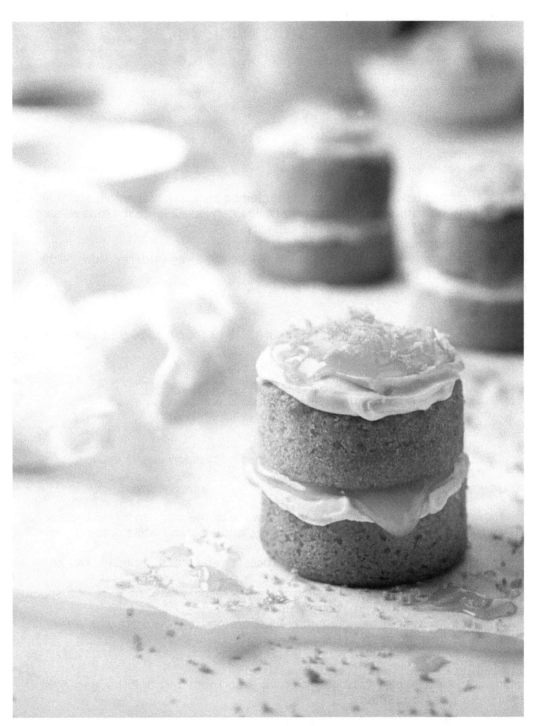

Lemon Curd Mini Cake

Prep time: 10 minutes | Cook time: 2 minutes | Makes 2

- ¼ cup plus 2 tablespoons all-purpose flour
- ½ teaspoon baking powder
- Pinch of salt
- 1 egg, beaten
- Zest of ¼ lemon
- 2 tablespoons granulated sweetener
- 2 tablespoons vegetable oil
- ¼ cup plus 2 tablespoons low-fat milk
- 2 teaspoons lemon curd

1. Put the flour, baking powder, salt, egg, lemon zest, sweetener, oil, and milk in a bowl and stir well until smooth. Divide between 2 large microwave-safe mugs or cups (with about ²/₃ cup capacity).
2. Cook in the microwave for 2 minutes.
3. Let cool for a few minutes. The cakes will shrink away from the sides of the cup. Top with the lemon curd.
4. Serve warm.

Per Serving

calories: 453 | total carbs: 27.9g | protein: 25.2g | total fat: 26.9g | sugar: 4.8g fiber: 3.3g | sodium: 176mg

Cheesy Berry Compote

Prep time: 10 minutes | Cook time: 0 minutes | Serves 4

- 1¼ cups blackberries
- 1¼ cups raspberries
- 1 tablespoon confectioners' sugar
- 1 tablespoons water
- 8 ounces (227 g) ricotta
- 1 teaspoon vanilla extract
- 2 graham crackers, crushed
- Mint sprigs, for garnish

1. Halve the blackberries and place in a bowl with the raspberries, sweetener, and water. Stir well to crush very slightly, and let stand while preparing the ricotta.
2. Put the ricotta and vanilla in a food processor and blend until smooth and creamy.
3. Divide the ricotta between serving plates, spreading with the back of a spoon. Pile the fruits on top with their syrup.
4. Scatter with the crushed graham cracker crumbs and decorate with a few sprigs of fresh mints to serve.

Per Serving

calories: 152 | total carbs: 12.4g | protein: 7.6g | total fat: 8.3g | sugar: 5.0g fiber: 4.9g | sodium: 60mg

Berry, Mango, and Kiwi Cake

Prep time: 5 minutes | Cook time: 0 minutes | Serves 6

- 8 ounces (227 g) frozen mixed berries
- 1 pound (454 g) fat-free plain Greek yogurt, divided
- 2 tablespoons granulated

- sweetener, divided
- 8 ounces (227 g) mango, chopped
- 11 ounces (312 g) kiwi fruit, chopped

1. Put a quarter of the frozen berries on the bottom of a loaf pan.
2. Blend the remainder of the berries with 6 ounces (142 g) of the yogurt and 1 tablespoon of the sweetener. Spread over the berries in the pan and freeze for 1½ hours.
3. Blend the mango with 7 ounces (198 g) of the yogurt and spread over the berry layer. Freeze for another 1 hour, until solid.
4. Blend the kiwi with the remaining yogurt and sweetener and spread over the mango layer. Cover with plastic wrap and freeze for 2 hours.
5. To serve, turn out onto a plate, wait for 15 minutes to allow the cake to soften, then slice to serve.

Per Serving

calories: 114 | total carbs: 19.5g | protein: 8.5g | total fat: 0.5g | sugar: 17.3g
fiber: 1.0g | sodium: 29mg

Super Easy Chocolate Mousse

Prep time: 5 minutes | Cook time: 0 minutes | Serves 4

- 4 ounces (113 g) chocolate, broken up
- 4 eggs, separated

1. Melt the chocolate in a bowl over boiling water, or in the microwave, and let cool, until barely warm.
2. Add the egg yolks to the chocolate and mix well.
3. Whisk the egg whites in a clean bowl until they stand in stiff peaks. Fold into the chocolate mixture with a metal spoon. Spoon into glasses and chill to set, about 2 to 3 hours.

Per Serving

calories: 245 | total carbs: 8.4g | protein: 9.6g | total fat: 19.0g | sugar: 0.4g
fiber: 4.7g | sodium: 69mg

Fig and Orange Cheesecake

Prep time: 15 minutes | Cook time: 35 minutes | Serves 8

- ¼ cup butter
- 2½ tablespoons honey
- 1⅔ cups oats
- 1¾ cups low-fat cream cheese, softened
- 3 eggs, separated
- ¼ cup plus 2 tablespoons granulated sweetener
- 1 teaspoon vanilla extract
- 4 ripe figs
- 2 oranges, peeled, pith removed, and sliced crosswise
- 2 tablespoons no-added-sugar apricot jam
- 2 tablespoons ginger wine, warmed

1. Preheat the oven to 350°F (180°C).
2. Melt the butter and honey in a pan and then stir in the oats, mixing well. Press into the bottom of a nonstick springform cake pan.
3. Whisk the cream cheese with the egg yolks, sweetener, and vanilla, until smooth.
4. Whisk the egg whites until stiff, then fold into the cream cheese mixture. Pour onto the cheesecake crust.
5. Bake for 35 to 40 minutes, or until golden and just firm to the touch. Let cool before removing from the pan and transferring to a serving plate.
6. Cut the figs into thin slices and place them on top of the cheesecake, overlapping them in a circular pattern with the orange slices. Mix the apricot jam with the ginger wine to make a glaze, and brush over the figs. Chill to serve.

Per Serving

calories: 437 | total carbs: 52.8g | protein: 13.7g | total fat: 19.8g | sugar: 19.4g fiber: 7.7g | sodium: 253mg

Gelatin Cottage Cheese

Prep time: 5 minutes | Cook time: 0 minutes | Serves 4

- 2 (24-ounce / 680-g) containers fat-free Cottage cheese
- 1 (8-ounce / 227-g) container
- sugar-free whipped topping
- 2 (3-ounce / 85-g) packages sugar-free gelatin

1. Mix all the ingredients in a big bowl.
2. Serve immediately.

Per Serving

calories: 97.8 | total carbs: 7.8g | protein: 13.7g | total fat: 1.1g | sugar: 5.4g fiber: 0g | sodium: 611mg

Peanut Butter Oat Cookies

Prep time: 10 minutes | Cook time: 8 minutes | Makes 18 cookies

- 1 cup unsweetened peanut butter
- 1 cup Splenda
- 1 egg
- 1 teaspoon vanilla
- 1 cup quick oats
- ½ teaspoon cinnamon, dried

1. Preheat the oven to 350ºF (180ºC).
2. Put the peanut butter and Splenda in a mixing bowl. Beat until smooth.
3. Whisk the egg and vanilla in the mixture. Fold in the oats and cinnamon. Continue to mix until the dough is sanity.
4. Scoop the dough out with a spoon and roll the dough into balls. Put the balls on a cookie sheet and squish them gently down with a fork.
5. Put cookies in the oven and bake for 8 minutes until golden brown.
6. Allow to cool before serving.

Per Serving (1 cookie)
calories: 6 | total carbs: 1.0g | protein: 0.2g | total fat: 0.2g | sugar: 0.7g
fiber: 0.1g | sodium: 13mg

Rhubarb Apple Popsicles

Prep time: 10 minutes | Cook time: 0 minutes | Makes 4 popsicles

- 2 cups rhubarb, diced
- 1 cup applesauce, unsweetened
- 2 teaspoons agave syrup or sugar

1. Put the rhubarb slices and a little water in a saucepan over medium heat. Cover and cook while occasionally stirring until it becomes a mush.
2. Remove from heat and stir in the applesauce and syrup.
3. Ladle the mixture into Popsicle forms. Put in the freezer to set. Serve chilled.

Per Serving (1 popsicle)
calories: 48 | total carbs: 12.4g | protein: 0.7g | total fat: 0.2g | sugar: 9.1g
fiber: 1.8g | sodium: 6mg

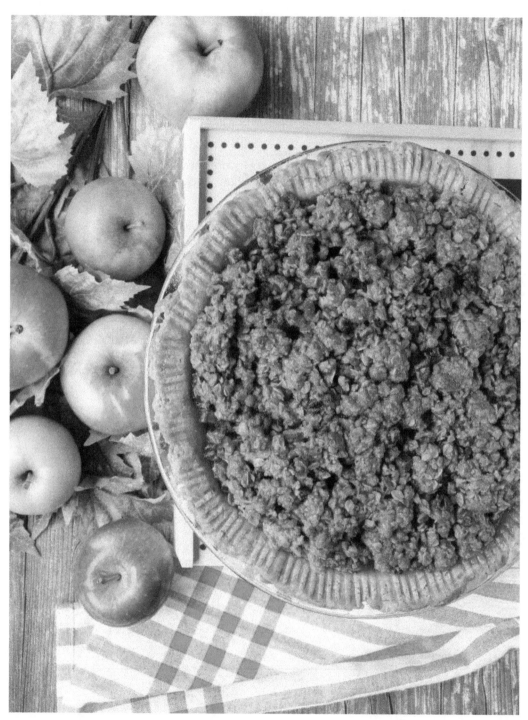

Toffee Apple Protein Crumble

Prep time: 15 minutes | Cook time: 10 minutes | Serves 4

- 3 large apples, peeled, cored, and chopped
- 1½ teaspoons low-sugar fruit syrup
- ¼ teaspoon ground cinnamon
- ½ teaspoon coconut oil
- Juice of ½ small orange

For the Protein Crumble Topping:

- 1 ounce (28 g) vanilla protein powder
- 1 cup oats
- ¼ cup ground almonds
- 2 tablespoons coconut oil
- 1½ teaspoons low-sugar fruit syrup

1. Preheat the oven to 325°F (170°C).
2. Put the apples, syrup, cinnamon, coconut oil, and orange juice in a large pan and cook, until the liquid starts to caramelize and the apples soften. Spoon into a baking dish.
3. Meanwhile, mix the protein powder with the oats and ground almonds. Add the coconut oil and fruit syrup, and rub together with the fingertips to make a light crumble topping. Sprinkle on top of the apple base.
4. Bake until the crumble topping is lightly browned, about 5 minutes.
5. Serve warm.

Per Serving
calories: 291 | total carbs: 42.9g | protein: 10.0g | total fat: 14.6g | sugar: 18.8g
fiber: 9.0g | sodium: 23mg

Chapter 14

Dressings, Sauces, and Seasonings

130   Caesar Dressing

130   Lemony Yogurt Sauce

131   Ranch Dressing

131   Taco Seasoning

132   Cajun Seasoning

132   Tonnato Sauce

133   Shallot Satay Sauce

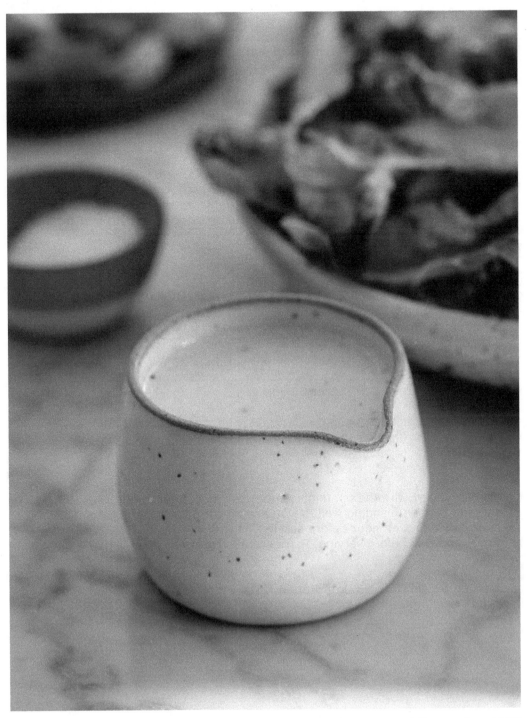

Caesar Dressing

Prep time: 10 minutes | Cook time: 0 minutes | Makes 1 cup

- ½ cup low-fat plain Greek yogurt
- ½ cup shredded Parmesan cheese
- ¼ cup freshly squeezed lemon juice
- ¼ cup low-fat milk
- 1 tablespoon extra-virgin olive oil
- 2 anchovy fillets, jarred or canned
- 2 teaspoons Worcestershire sauce
- 1 teaspoon minced garlic
- 1 teaspoon Dijon mustard
- 1 teaspoon onion powder
- ½ teaspoon freshly ground black pepper

1. In a blender or food processor, purée the yogurt, cheese, lemon juice, milk, olive oil, anchovies, Worcestershire sauce, garlic, mustard, onion powder, and pepper on medium-high speed until the dressing is smooth and creamy without any lumps.
2. Serve immediately.

Per Serving (2 tablespoons)
calories: 62 | total carbs: 3.5g | protein: 3.2g | total fat: 4.0g | sugar: 1.8g
fiber: 0.8g | sodium: 185mg

Lemony Yogurt Sauce

Prep time: 5 minutes | Cook time: 0 minutes | Serves 8

- 2 cups whole-milk plain yogurt
- ¼ cup extra virgin olive oil
- ½ cup finely chopped fresh mint
- 1 teaspoon grated lemon zest
- 1 tablespoon lemon juice
- Salt and freshly ground black pepper, to taste

1. Mix the yogurt with the oil, mint, lemon zest, lemon juice, and season with salt and pepper, blending well. If you are preparing in advance, do not add the mint until about an hour before serving.
2. Cover and chill before serving. Refrigerate leftovers and use within 2 days.

Per Serving
calories: 97 | total carbs: 3.0g | protein: 2.1g | total fat: 8.8g | sugar: 2.9g
fiber: 0g | sodium: 28mg

Ranch Dressing

Prep time: 10 minutes | Cook time: 0 minutes | Serves 15

- ⅔ cup skim milk
- 2 teaspoons white wine vinegar
- ⅔ cup extra-light mayonnaise
- ½ teaspoon garlic powder
- ¼ teaspoon onion powder
- 1 teaspoon mustard powder
- 1 teaspoon chopped fresh parsley
- 4 scallions, finely chopped or ¼ cup snipped fresh chives
- Salt and freshly ground black pepper, to taste

1. Mix the milk with the vinegar in a bowl and allow to stand for 10 minutes.
2. Whisk the milk mixture with the mayonnaise, and the garlic, onion, and mustard powders, until smooth.
3. Add the parsley, scallions, and salt and pepper. Cover and chill, to thicken slightly. The dressing will improve and become more flavorful as it keeps.

Per Serving
calories: 43 | total carbs: 2.5g | protein: 0.6g | total fat: 3.4g | sugar: 1.9g
fiber: 0.1g | sodium: 84mg

Taco Seasoning

Prep time: 5 minutes | Cook time: 0 minutes | Makes: 2½ tablespoons

- ¾ teaspoon garlic powder
- ½ teaspoon onion powder
- ¼ teaspoon red pepper flakes
- ¾ teaspoon dried oregano
- 2 teaspoons ground paprika
- 1 teaspoon freshly ground black pepper
- 2 teaspoons ground cumin
- ½ teaspoon ground cayenne pepper

1. In a container with an airtight lid, combine the garlic powder, onion powder, red pepper flakes, oregano, paprika, black pepper, cumin, and cayenne pepper. Put the lid on, give the container a few shakes.

Per Serving (2½ tablespoons)
calories: 44 | total carbs: 7.9g | protein: 2.1g | total fat: 1.6g | sugar: 0.9g
fiber: 2.8g | sodium: 13mg

Cajun Seasoning

Prep time: 5 minutes | Cook time: 0 minutes | Makes 3½ tablespoons

- 1½ tablespoons ground paprika
- 1½ teaspoons onion powder
- 1½ teaspoons garlic powder
- ½ teaspoon freshly ground black pepper
- 1 teaspoon ground cayenne pepper
- ½ teaspoon ground cumin
- ½ teaspoon dried thyme
- ½ teaspoon dried oregano

1. In a container with an airtight lid, combine the paprika, onion powder, garlic powder, black pepper, cayenne pepper, cumin, thyme, and oregano. Put the lid on, give the container a few shakes.

Per Serving (3½ tablespoons)
calories: 69 | total carbs: 14.0g | protein: 3.1g | total fat: 2.0g | sugar: 1.7g fiber: 5.5g | sodium: 15mg

Tonnato Sauce

Prep time: 10 minutes | Cook time: 10 minutes | Serves 6

- 8 ounces (225 g) tuna in oil, drained (reserve 1 tablespoon oil)
- 3 anchovy fillets
- ¾ cup light mayonnaise
- 2 teaspoons Dijon mustard
- 1 tablespoon lemon juice
- Salt and freshly ground black pepper, to taste

2. Put the tuna and the reserved oil in a food processor or blender with the anchovies, mayonnaise, mustard, lemon juice, 1 tablespoon water, and season with salt and pepper. Blend until smooth.
3. Check the consistency of the mixture. It should be like a custard sauce—if necessary, add an additional tablespoon water and blend again.
4. Use to coat cooked and sliced chicken or turkey, or as a dip or sauce for cooked or crisp vegetables.

Per Serving
calories: 436 | total carbs: 2.2g | protein: 0.9g | total fat: 47.7g | sugar: 1.3g fiber: 0.1g | sodium: 304mg

Shallot Satay Sauce

Prep time: 10 minutes | Cook time: 10 minutes | Serves 8

- 2 teaspoons sesame oil
- 3 shallots, roughly chopped
- 1 tablespoon curry paste
- 3 tablespoons smooth no-added-
- sugar peanut butter
- 5 ounces (142 g) coconut cream
- Juice of 1 lime

1. Heat the oil in a small pan, add the shallots, and cook gently for 4 minutes, until they soften.
2. Stir in the curry paste, peanut butter, coconut cream, and lime juice, mixing well.
3. Bring to a simmer and cook for 6 minutes until the sauce has thickened, then blend with an immersion blender until smooth.
4. Serve warm.

Per Serving

calories: 115 | total carbs: 6.3g | protein: 2.8g | total fat: 9.7g | sugar: 1.6g
fiber: 1.5g | sodium: 39mg

Appendix 1 Measurement Conversion Chart

VOLUME EQUIVALENTS(DRY)

US STANDARD	METRIC (APPROXIMATE)
1/8 teaspoon	0.5 mL
1/4 teaspoon	1 mL
1/2 teaspoon	2 mL
3/4 teaspoon	4 mL
1 teaspoon	5 mL
1 tablespoon	15 mL
1/4 cup	59 mL
1/2 cup	118 mL
3/4 cup	177 mL
1 cup	235 mL
2 cups	475 mL
3 cups	700 mL
4 cups	1 L

VOLUME EQUIVALENTS(LIQUID)

US STANDARD	US STANDARD (OUNCES)	METRIC (APPROXIMATE)
2 tablespoons	1 fl.oz.	30 mL
1/4 cup	2 fl.oz.	60 mL
1/2 cup	4 fl.oz.	120 mL
1 cup	8 fl.oz.	240 mL
1 1/2 cup	12 fl.oz.	355 mL
2 cups or 1 pint	16 fl.oz.	475 mL
4 cups or 1 quart	32 fl.oz.	1 L
1 gallon	128 fl.oz.	4 L

TEMPERATURES EQUIVALENTS

FAHRENHEIT(F)	CELSIUS(C) (APPROXIMATE)
225 °F	107 °C
250 °F	120 °C
275 °F	135 °C
300 °F	150 °C
325 °F	160 °C
350 °F	180 °C
375 °F	190 °C
400 °F	205 °C
425 °F	220 °C
450 °F	235 °C
475 °F	245 °C
500 °F	260 °C

WEIGHT EQUIVALENTS

US STANDARD	METRIC (APPROXIMATE)
1 ounce	28 g
2 ounces	57 g
5 ounces	142 g
10 ounces	284 g
15 ounces	425 g
16 ounces (1 pound)	455 g
1.5 pounds	680 g
2 pounds	907 g

Appendix 2 Recipe Index

A

Adobo Black Bean Hummus 76
Almond and Cherry Shake 40
Apple Braised Pork 111
Artichoke and Spinach Chicken Rolls102
Avocado and Egg Toast 66
Avocado Milk Whip 48
Avocado Turkey Blt 105

B

Baked Oatmeal with Cherries and Apple 70
Banana and Kale Smoothie 49
BBQ Chicken with Avocado 106
Beef and mushroom Stroganoff 111
Beef Bone Broth 41
Beef Brisket Roast 113
Beef Purée 53
Berries and Walnut Pops 58
Berry, Mango, and Kiwi Cake 119
Blueberry and Spinach Smoothie 50
Broccoli Purée 48
Butternut Squash and Cauliflower Hash Browns 71

C

Caesar Dressing 126
Cajun Seasoning 128
Caprese Skewers 75
Cauliflower and Shrimp Chowder 94
Cauliflower Mash 77
Cheesy Berry Compote 118
Chia Protein Oatmeal 59
Chicken and Water Chestnut Wraps 106
Chicken Bone and Vegetable Broth 45
Chocolate and Peanut Smoothie 42
Cod en Papillote 99
Coffee Protein Shake 42
Creamy Banana Shake 44

Creamy Broccoli Soup 84
Creamy Cheese Berry Smoothies 59
Creamy Chicken and Vegetable Soup 63
Creamy Egg and Tuna Salad 58
Creamy Horseradish London Broil 110
Creamy Parmesan and Dill Halibut 95
Cucumber and Tomato Salad 79
Cucumber Turkey Rolls 107

D-E

Deviled Eggs 75
Easy Chocolate and Orange Pudding 49

F-G

Fig and Orange Cheesecake 120
Garden Vegetable Roast 77
Gelatin Cottage Cheese 120

H

Hearty Beef Bordelaise 115
Hearty Gazpacho 57
Herbed Chicken Purée 54

L

Lemon Curd Mini Cake 118
Lemony Sole 95
Lemony Yogurt Sauce 126
Lush Pumpkin Smoothie 40
Lush Roasted Vegetable Salad 85

M-O

Madeira Pork Tenderloin 112
Mango and Banana Porridge 57
Matcha Mango Smoothie 50
Mexican Salsa Chicken 107
Mini Egg White Pizza 67
Oat and Fruit Smoothie 61

P

Peanut Butter Oat Cookies   121
Pork Medallions with Mushrooms   112
Pork Tenderloin Asian Style   110
Pumpkin and Zucchini Muffins   72
Puréed Strawberries with Creamy Yogurt   62

R

Radish Chips   76
Ranch Dressing   127
Rhubarb Apple Popsicles   121
Ricotta Peach Fluff   50
Ritzy Beef and Veg Stir-fry   114

S

Salmon Crackers   94
Salsa Verde Chicken Bowl   103
Scallops with Broccoli   96
Scrambled Eggs   61
Seitan Bites   86
Shallot Satay Sauce   129
Shrimp and Vegetable Salad   97
Simple Applesauce   52
Simple Cottage Pancakes   67
Simple Salmon Roast   97
Sloppy Joes in Lettuce   88
Southwest Egg and Vegetable Scramble   66
Spaghetti Squash Noodles   87
Spinach Dip   79
Spinach Quiche   68
Split Pea and Carrot Soup   52
Strawberry Crème Shake   44
Super Easy Chocolate Mousse   119
Super Skim Milk   41
Super Veg Chili   83

T

Taco Seasoning   127
Tempeh and Avocado Lettuce Wraps   89
Tempeh, Mushroom and Broccoli Bowl   83
Toffee Apple Protein Crumble   123
Tomato Scrambled Egg with Bacon   62
Tonnato Sauce   128
Tuna and Apple Salad   96
Turkey and Spinach Burgers   105

V

Veg and Chicken Meatballs   104
Vegetable Deli Turkey Rolls   80

Y

Yogurt and Mixed Berry Crumble   68

Z

Zoodles with "Meat" Sauce   91
Zucchini Fries   80